JMA]

POSITIVE DENTAL PREVENTION

The prevention in childhood of dental disease in adult life

POSITIVE DENTAL PREVENTION

The prevention in childhood of dental disease in adult life

Edited by

Richard J. Elderton BDS, PhD
*Professor of Preventive and Restorative Dentistry
Department of Conservative Dentistry
University of Bristol*

HEINEMANN MEDICAL BOOKS

Heinemann Medical Books
An imprint of Heinemann Professional Publishing Ltd
Halley Court, Jordan Hill, Oxford OX2 8EJ

OXFORD   LONDON   SINGAPORE   NAIROBI
IBADAN   KINGSTON

First published in 1987
Reprinted 1989

British Library Cataloguing in Publication Data

Positive Dental Prevention:
Prevention in childhood of dental disease in adult life.
  1. Children—Dental care—Great Britain
  I. Elderton, Richard J.
  617.6'01'088054   RK55.C5

ISBN 0 433 00018 X

Typeset by D. P. Media Limited, Hitchin, Hertfordshire.
Printed and bound in Great Britain by Redwood Burn Ltd, Trowbridge

Contents

Foreword

One of the most important functions of the Community Dental Services Group of the British Dental Association is to support and foster postgraduate study. This it has done over many years by organising courses, usually two each year, on subjects especially appropriate to the needs of dentists working in the community dental services.

The Group invited Professor Richard Elderton of the University of Bristol Dental School to plan and organise the content of its 1987 autumn postgraduate course at the University of East Anglia. His enthusiastic response to this approach, and his collaboration with the Group's Postgraduate Committee, led to a wide-ranging course entitled *Prevention in Childhood of Dental Disease in Adult Life*. Further to that, following Professor Elderton's suggestion, the Group decided that there should be a publication to accompany the course, and that this should subsequently be made available to interested individuals and organisations. By this means, an event into which much thought and work had gone, would be recorded permanently and reach a wider audience.

The Community Dental Services Group is confident that the quality of the contributions and the range of topics covered will ensure that the publication is a most valuable one.

G. J. Tucker   *September, 1987*
President
Community Dental Services Group
of the British Dental Association

Preface

Dentistry is changing. The prevention of most dental disease is a realistic possibility today in the UK and in other countries where caries levels have fallen in recent years. In many developing countries, where caries levels are currently rising, it may, however, be some time before this sense of optimism can prevail; but this should in no way inhibit the implementation of up-to-date preventive measures in these countries.

Has preventive dentistry become rather a tired message? Do we now 'know it all'? I think not. Preventive dentistry has come of age and horizons have stretched to embrace a wider range of endeavour than has sometimes been the case in the past.

Where better to start prevention than with the child—and with the long-term aim of helping the child to become a dentally healthy adult with the least need for a lifetime of interventive and maintenance dental treatment? Hence the title of this book: *Positive Dental Prevention: the prevention in childhood of dental disease in adult life.*

This is essentially a practical book, for prevention is a practical subject and it only works if it is applied. But before preventive measures are discussed, Chapter 1 sets the scene, while Chapters 2–4 examine current understanding about the processes of periodontal disease and dental caries, together with their detection and assessment. The widespread nature of periodontal disease in children is stressed, and the CPITN method of screening for the disease in children is described. Dental caries is discussed in terms of its dynamic nature, together with ways of identifying children at particular risk to its ravages. With the growing child in mind, Chapter 5 identifies the critical stages in development when screening should be undertaken for occlusal abnormalities, and provides guidelines as to action that should be taken by the general dentist when an abnormality is found. Chapters 6–8 discuss the preventive management of periodontal disease, together with diet, hygiene and fluoride considerations in the prevention and control of caries.

Chapters 9–13 are concerned with the important matter of restorative dentistry, addressing major problems in this area that are now looming large on the dental scene, including: shortcomings in the diagnosis and planning of restorative treatment; problems with restoratively-orientated dental care in general, and problems with outdated restorations and restorative procedures in particular. This leads into the preventive management of dental caries using techniques which require the least amount of invasive intervention. But as restorations and sealant restorations will still be required for the foreseeable future, preventively-orientated cavity design and restorative procedures are described in Chapter 12.

In patients with developing dentitions, elective, correctly-timed extractions should sometimes be undertaken as a powerful preventive measure for the good of the dentition as a whole and in the interests of long-term dental health. Chapter 14 explains the technique of serial extractions and considers the management of deciduous and permanent molars with a poor restorative prognosis. The circumstances that dictate the need for balancing and compensating extractions are discussed, together with the preventive management of the occlusion when permanent teeth are developmentally absent.

With the general dentist increasingly becoming involved in the management of the developing dentition, the place which myofunctional appliances occupy in interceptive orthodontics forms the subject of Chapter 15, particular reference being made to their role in the management of patients with prominent upper incisors. In spite of preventive measures that might be taken, these teeth are sometimes knocked out traumatically, in which case a satisfactory long-term outcome is very dependent upon the way the dentist manages the child at the time. The prevention of this unfortunate accident, first aid measures that should be taken if it occurs, replantation, and the assessment of the patient for long-term treatment planning, form the subject of Chapter 16. Crowding in the dentition after the eruption of the second permanent molars, is discussed in Chapter 17.

This book considers the child from the cradle to adulthood with respect to a developing dentition which is potentially subject to the common dental diseases. The dentist who looks after the child has a responsibility not only to help him or her to effect relevant preventive measures, but also to enact a preventive philosophy in the management of any conditions that may arise. In this way, prevention in childhood really can lead to dental health in adult life.

Richard J. Elderton   *September, 1987*

Contributors

R. J. ANDLAW LDSRCS, MSc, PhD
Consultant Senior Lecturer
Department of Child Dental Health
University of Bristol Dental School
Bristol

A. S. BLINKHORN BDS, MSc, PhD
Consultant in Paediatric Dentistry
Department of Child Dental Health
Glasgow Dental Hospital and Royal Hospital for Sick Children
Glasgow

I. D. BROWN BDS, FDS, DOrth, PhD
Lecturer in Orthodontics
Department of Child Dental Health
University of Bristol Dental School
Bristol

R. J. ELDERTON BDS, PhD
Professor of Preventive and Restorative Dentistry
Department of Conservative Dentistry
University of Bristol Dental School
Bristol

D. A. M. GEDDES BDS, MSc, FDS, PhD
Senior Lecturer in Preventive Dentistry and Periodontology
Head of Oral Biology Group
University of Glasgow Dental Hospital and School
Glasgow

J. LUKER BDS, FDS
Research Associate
University Department of Oral Medicine, Oral Surgery and Pathology
University of Bristol Dental School
Bristol

J. J. MURRAY MChD, FDS, PhD
Professor of Child Dental Health
Department of Child Dental Health
University of Newcastle upon Tyne Dental School
Newcastle upon Tyne

C. D. STEPHENS MDS, FDS, DOrth
Professor of Child Dental Health
Department of Child Dental Health
University of Bristol Dental School
Bristol

Colour Plates

Plate 1 *The anterior dentition and periodontium of an 11-year-old boy. Note the plaque accumulation around the gingival margins and the prominence of the interdental papillae between the upper left central and lateral incisors, which are red and swollen and which bled profusely after probing. This young boy has gingivitis which can be expected to resolve if the plaque deposits are removed and the patient prevents their return by careful, efficient toothbrushing.*

Plate 2 *Upper second molar with clearly visible white spot caries in the sides of the occlusal fissure. Only the eye can make this diagnosis. Fissure sealant was applied as a therapeutic treatment. (Reproduced by kind permission of A.E. Morgan, Publishers of Restorative Dentistry.)*

Plate 3 *Upper premolar in a 14-year-old child showing the development of brown discolouration associated with caries in the fissure. Visualisation of such lesions is imperative. Fissure sealant was applied.*

Plate 4 *Large arrested dentine caries lesions in a 5-year-old child for whom a preventive programme has now worked. Note the loss of deciduous molars that took place earlier when the disease was active.*

Plate 5 *Anterior view of the teeth of a 4-year-old boy who had had prolonged use of a sugar comforter. A change of diet alone enabled the progression of caries in the upper incisors to be halted. This dietary advice to the family resulted in freedom from caries in the second child.*

Plate 6 *Fissure sealed lower molar in a 12-year-old. The defect at the distal edge of the sealant could result in the initiation of caries; and it could result in an invasive restorative procedure (which might not be warranted). If the tooth had not been sealed, it might have remained both caries-free and restoration-free.*

Plate 7 *Plaque-covered first permanent molar in an 8-year-old child. The tooth cannot be assessed until it has been cleaned, and it would be naive to think the child or parent could be taught to clean the tooth effectively every day. See Plate 8.*

Plate 8 *The tooth shown in Plate 7 after cleaning with pumice. Early white spot caries can now be seen in the centre of the fissure system. Fissure sealant was applied.*

Plate 9 *Lower molar with an occlusal carious lesion centred on the lingual fissure. A radiograph revealed the existence of definite dentine involvement, a feature suggested by the dark hue shining through the surrounding enamel. But the true extent of the lesion was unknown. The affected pit is in a relatively unprotected site. All these features led to the decision to excise the lesion and restore, rather than to treat with fissure sealant. (See also Fig. 12.4, p.87).*

Plate 10 *Example of a lower first permanent molar with a relatively poor long-term prognosis. The extensive occlusal restoration involving the disto-lingual cusp, together with the lingual restoration and associated plaque, make the tooth ripe for (passive) entry into a cycle of repeat restorations. Proper occlusal assessment of patients with first molars like this, with a view to their extraction (together with balancing and/or compensating extractions as appropriate) is a valuable aspect of prevention in childhood of dental disease in adult life. But having extracted them, it behoves the dentist to put in hand active preventive management of the premolars and second molars.*

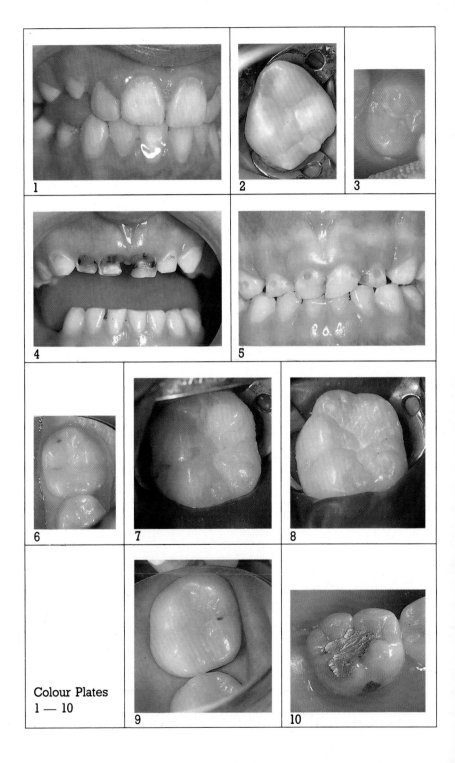

Colour Plates
1 — 10

1

The Potential for Prevention in Children

J. J. MURRAY

Levels of dental caries have risen in many developing parts of the world in recent years, yet they have fallen in many industrialised countries. The best chronicles of change in the dental health of children in England and Wales are the national surveys of Children's Dental Health in 1973[1] and in 1983[2]. This latter survey also included Scotland and Northern Ireland.

DENTAL CARIES

The proportion of 5-year-olds with caries has declined from 72% in 1973 to 49% in 1983; and the dmf has fallen from 4.0 to 1.8. The resulting increased retention of deciduous molars appears to explain a discernible trend for premolars to be erupting slightly later now than in 1973.

A reduction of about 30% has been observed in caries in the permanent dentition. Thus the mean DMF in 15-year-olds fell from 8.4 to 5.6 over the 10-year period. However, considering the whole of the UK, only 9% of children in 1983 had no evidence of caries experience or restorations in any of their first permanent molars; indeed, 62% had evidence of one or the other in all four of these teeth. Obviously, this general trend is a most welcome development but there is a long way to go. Caries prevalence in children should be considered to have fallen from very high levels to medium levels. The most important objective now is to develop strategies which favour further caries prevention and which identify and direct treatment to those subgroups within the population which still have a high caries experience (*see* Chapter 2, p. 7).

PERIODONTAL DISEASE

The 1983 survey revealed that about half of all children had periodontal inflammation, this rising from 19% among 5-year-olds, to 50% of the 9-year-old and older age groups. Using the World Health Organization 621 probe, 48% of 15-year-olds were found to have gingivitis (identified by bleeding following probing). Periodontal pocketing was found in 9%, though in less than 1 in 200 of 15-year-olds was there pocketing of 5.5 mm or more. However, this means the average secondary school will have one or more of these individuals within its ranks.

The proportions of children with calculus and periodontal disease did not change greatly in England and Wales between 1973 and 1983, though plaque, calculus and inflammation levels appear to have fallen slightly. It is clear that greater emphasis needs to be directed to this area of dental care.

OCCLUSION

In the 1983 Survey it was found that nearly three-quarters of the children examined with respect to orthodontic criteria had one or more of the following conditions (though not necessarily requiring treatment):

- crowding;
- an overjet of 5 mm or more;
- an incisor that was rotated, instanding or in an edge-to-edge relationship;
- traumatic injury due to an increased overbite.

The 9-year-old age group showed the highest proportion with some orthodontic need; 47% were considered to need treatment for crowding, and 16% for overjet reduction. Among the children aged 12, 20% had received some orthodontic treatment, a figure which rose to one-third by the age of 15. It was estimated that a quarter of 14-year-olds and a fifth of 15-year-olds had not had orthodontic treatment and needed it.

The proportion of children in England and Wales who had had orthodontic extractions or appliance therapy rose slightly between 1973 and 1983, though the proportion of children considered to be in need of orthodontic treatment had not changed significantly during the 10-year period.

ACCIDENTAL DAMAGE TO INCISORS

By the age of 15 years, 33% of boys and 19% of girls in the 1983 survey had suffered damage to at least one incisor tooth. Regrettably, in 84% of cases, this damage remained untreated, though in many instances the damage was limited to fracturing of the enamel.

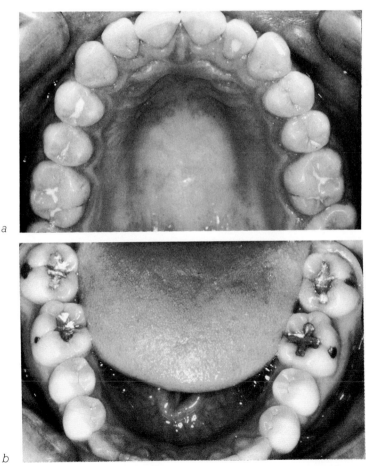

a

b

Fig. 1.1a and **b** a = *Occlusal view of the maxillary arch of teeth in a 17-year-old girl showing fissure sealants in place. b = Occlusal view of the mandibular arch showing occlusal and buccal amalgams in the permanent molars.*

PROSPECTS FOR ADULTHOOD

It may be a gross simplification and generalisation to say that by
the age of 12–14 years the future dental treatment needs of a
patient are largely determined, but this may often be the case.
Consider the dental condition of the patient illustrated in Fig. 1.1*a*
and *b* (p. 3). She has a beautiful smile and good oral hygiene. Her
upper arch shows true prevention, with all four permanent molars
fissure-sealed. The lower arch has been preserved by amalgam
restorations in the occlusal and buccal surfaces. Which arch will

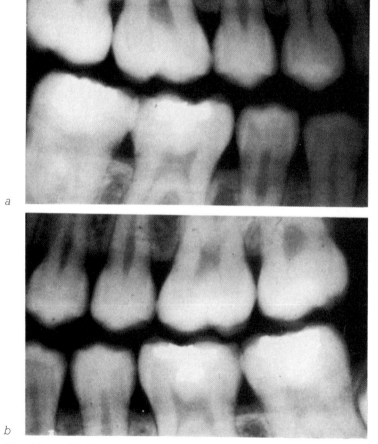

a

b

Fig. 1.2a and **b** *Bitewing radiographs of the patient shown in Fig. 1.1.*

require further dental attention in future years? How often will these amalgams be replaced and extended in the next 50 years? Why was caries prevented in the upper arch but excised and the teeth restored in the lower arch? The bitewing radiographs certainly suggest that some of the occlusal amalgams are minimal and that they might have been obviated by a more preventive approach (Fig. 1.2*a* and *b*).

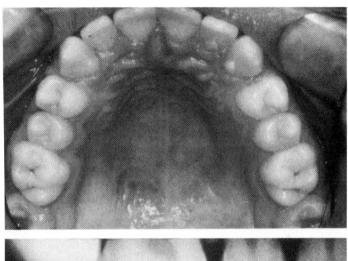

a

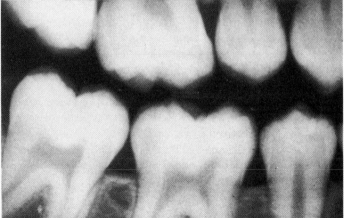

b

Fig. 1.3a and ***b*** *a* = Occlusal view of the upper arch of a 13-year-old patient, showing staining in the fissures of the first permanent molars. The lower teeth were the same. All these fissures were sealed at the age of 7. b = Right bitewing radiograph of this patient. The left radiograph revealed a similar lack of disease.

When the earliest signs of decalcification are observed in first permanent molars soon after they erupt, it is very easy to feel that the patient is particularly caries-susceptible. However, by fissure sealing these teeth and paying proper attention to oral hygiene and diet control, amalgam and other restorations can be avoided, as seen in the child shown in Fig. 1.3*a* and *b* (p. 5). At 13 years of age, and with the permanent teeth in occlusion, radiographs show the patient to be caries-free. With reasonable attention to preventive measures from this time onwards, it can be predicted that the patient will keep his teeth for life with no need for restorative treatment.

POTENTIAL FOR AN IMPROVED EPIDEMIOLOGICAL PICTURE

The dental profession has a responsibility for appreciating, and to a certain extent anticipating, changes that occur in the dental health of the nation. With two of the Oral Health Goals for the year 2000, set by the World Health Organization in 1980, already achieved in England (51% of 5-year-olds being caries-free and a mean DMF of 2.9 for 12-year-olds) there should be a general feeling of uplifting at the prospect of having within grasp the possibility that the current generation of children will have the lowest rate of tooth decay for over 100 years and that the disease really can be defeated. Of course, restorative skills will still be required, but the practice of dentistry must be allowed to develop in order to make the best use of new dental materials and techniques as they evolve. What is certain is that there is more time available now than formerly for implementing preventive measures against both caries and periodontal disease; for treating fractured and traumatised teeth; and for undertaking orthodontic assessments and treatment. There is now the potential for applying prevention in childhood with the real possibility of achieving dental health in adult life.

REFERENCES

1. Todd J. E. (1975). *Children's dental health in England and Wales 1973.* London: HMSO.
2. Todd J. E., Dodd T. (1985). *Children's dental health in the United Kingdom 1983.* London: HMSO.

2

Periodontal Disease and its Detection

J. LUKER

Periodontal disease is one of the most common bacterial conditions affecting mankind, though it is sometimes rather naively considered to concern only the adult population. It is clear from Chapter 1 that this is far from the truth. The sentiment does, however, reflect the paucity of published data concerning periodontal conditions in children and adolescents. The dentist should interact at an early stage in order to give these young people the maximum chance of entering adulthood with a healthy periodontium and be set on the road to maintaining this healthy status throughout adult life.

Periodontal disease is thought to be the result of a reaction of the host tissues to bacterial plaque, though in a few periodontal conditions it may be due to specific microorganisms within the plaque. Gingivitis, the earliest clinical sign of periodontal disease, can be seen, to a greater or lesser extent, in almost every individual with permanent teeth. However, the preschool child appears to have a reduced host immune response to plaque deposits, making gingivitis less common than in children at the mixed dentition stage, even with similar amounts of plaque deposit[1]. This may be due to an immature system or to a different oral flora in the very young.

If allowed to persist, gingivitis usually progresses to some irreversible loss of periodontal attachment, bone loss and eventually exfoliation of the teeth, a process which may take a lifetime or just a few years. There is considerable individual variability in the rate of progression of periodontal disease, some individuals being far more susceptible than others. These latter constitute an 'at-risk' group. The progression of periodontal disease is not continuous, there being periods of active progression and quiescence. In some instances, regression has been reported.

There is no doubt that plaque deposits adjacent to the gingival margin cause gingivitis, but the amount of plaque surrounding a tooth does not in itself provide a good indication of the extent of the periodontal disease. On the other hand, gingival bleeding following gentle probing, the presence of calculus deposits and pathological pockets (pockets which have their bases apical to the amelocemental junction) have been shown to correlate well with the disease process[2]. Bleeding from the gingival crevice or pocket is indicative of active disease, while a periodontal pocket which does not bleed after gentle probing may be considered to be quiescent; and it may remain so.

Susceptible individuals appear to react unfavourably to lower levels of plaque than do less susceptible individuals, and bleeding after probing in the presence of low plaque scores has been shown to be a good prognostic indicator[3]. Clearly it is important to use appropriate screening procedures to identify susceptible individuals.

The literature does not indicate a specific age at which irreversible periodontal destruction begins to take place. Certainly the onset of juvenile periodontitis is not usually considered to occur before 13–15 years of age. That the disease is not evident in younger children may reflect a lack of clinical data concerning the periodontal status, such as mobility and abcess formation, of affected individuals prior to the onset of advanced clinical manifestations. This itself may reflect inadequate periodontal screening.

SCREENING FOR PERIODONTAL DISEASE

Screening for any condition may be defined as a simple test for selecting out certain individuals from a group. It is, therefore, almost by definition, geared to populations, and it may therefore serve for the collection of epidemiological data as well as provide a basis for identifying patients who would benefit from a more detailed examination.

For effective primary prevention it would seem essential to screen for periodontal disease from as early as 7 years of age, which may be considered the age of onset of gingivitis[4]. At this age it is, of course, impossible to predict those individuals who are going to become particularly susceptible to periodontal disease. Periodontal conditions and treatment needs may be determined by clinical assessment of the presence or absence of the following:

- gingival swelling;
- bleeding from the gingiva (on probing);
- pathological pockets;
- calculus;
- incorrectly contoured restorations.

In young people, false pockets associated with normal tooth eruption often make it difficult to determine, by probing, whether periodontal disease is present or not. For subjects under 20 years of age, probing for pockets should, therefore, normally be restricted to the first permanent molars and the permanent incisors for, being the first permanent teeth to erupt, these are the least likely to have false pockets. They are also the most likely teeth to reveal any true periodontal breakdown at an early age.

Gingivitis associated with false pockets will be detected quite frequently and this can usually be treated by scaling and the institution of meticulous toothbrushing (*see* Chapter 6, p. 39 and Plate 1). Whether due to hyperplasia or to eruption, false pockets do not require treatment unless they exhibit gingival bleeding on probing.

CPITN FOR CHILDREN

The Community Periodontal Index of Treatment Needs (CPITN) assessment was established by the World Health Organization (WHO) in 1982, and is designed for rapid and practical assessment of treatment needs in population surveys and for initial screening of patients attending for dental care. Because children and adolescents have erupting and exfoliating teeth, the adult version of the CPITN index gives misleading results when applied to children. However, Ainamo *et al.*[5] undertook a study to determine how best to avoid such misleading CPITN recordings in people under 20 years old. These findings were incorporated into a simplified periodontal examination method for those aged 7–19 years based upon the CPITN[6]. This screening method is now described.

For the purposes of the index, just the four first permanent

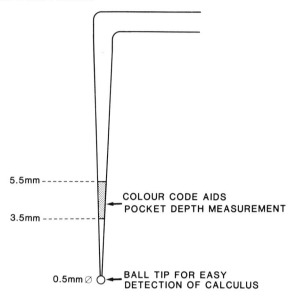

5.5mm ----------
3.5mm ----------

COLOUR CODE AIDS
POCKET DEPTH MEASUREMENT

0.5mm ⌀

BALL TIP FOR EASY
DETECTION OF CALCULUS

Fig. 2.1. *The 621 periodontal probe.*

molars and the maxillary right and mandibular left central incisors are included. When the designated tooth is missing, the sextant is scored as missing. The recommended examination instrument is the WHO periodontal probe (Fig. 2.1). The ball-ended feature of this instrument greatly helps in the detection of subgingival calculus or other roughness of the tooth surfaces and also facilitates the accurate assessment of the apical extent of any pockets, for it reduces the risk of overmeasurement. The colour coded region of the probe from 3.5–5.5 mm is intended to allow direct reading of pocket depths of 3 mm or less, pockets which are 4–5 mm deep, and pockets which are over 6 mm deep.

The probe is inserted carefully and gently between the tooth and gingiva, and the sulcus or pocket depth is observed against the colour code. The recommended probing force is between 12–25 g, and such probing should not cause pain or discomfort. The number of probings per index tooth is left to the discretion of the examiner. It is, however, usual for four areas to be examined per tooth: mesio-buccal; mesio-lingual; disto-buccal and disto-lingual. It should also be remembered that bleeding may not be observed during probing; rather, it may show up some 10–30 s after the probe has been withdrawn.

For those aged 11–19, the highest of the following codes for each index tooth is scored as follows:

Code 0   Healthy periodontal tissues.
Code 1   Gingival bleeding following gentle probing.
Code 2   Supra- or subgingival calculus or defective margin of restoration.
Code 3   Pathological pocket 4–5 mm deep.
Code 4   Pathological pocket 6 mm or deeper.

For those aged 7–11, it is recommended that only codes *1* and *2* are scored (on account of the likelihood of false pockets).

A simple box chart is used to record the appropriate scores, and an example is as follows:

3	2	4
4	3	3

Pockets of 6 mm or more (as in this example) in a child or adolescent are certainly indicative of high susceptibility to periodontal destruction, e.g. juvenile periodontitis or systemic predisposing factors, and the recording is sufficient to indicate referral of the patient to a specialist.

The scores are presumed to indicate the following periodontal treatment needs:

Code 0   No need for periodontal treatment.
Code 1   Oral hygiene instruction required.
Code 2   A need for scaling and root planing (including the
and 3   elimination of plaque-retentive margins of restorations and oral hygiene instruction).
Code 4   A need for complex treatment in addition to that for codes *2* and *3*.

Use of the modified CPITN should allow susceptible individuals to be identified as early as possible; certainly it will separate out those with juvenile periodontitis.

When used correctly, the modified CPITN fulfils the requirement of a screening procedure by providing quantifiable data for epidemiology and a basis for patient examination. It is also capable of selecting out those individuals who require a more detailed examination. This would normally include a CPITN assessment of each tooth and a thorough scan for predisposing causes. Should pathological pocket formation be recorded, alveolar bone levels should be checked using bitewing radiographs (Fig. 2.2). This allows the clinician to:

- confirm the diagnosis;
- assess more clearly the amount of bone loss;
- make subsequent comparisons in order to assess any progression of the lesion.

The CPITN may serve also to trigger a specialist periodontal consultation or orthodontic assessment and, occasionally, medical referral will be indicated.

It should be appreciated that as only six teeth are used for the screening procedure, localised periodontal problems, which may include high fraenal attachments, fenestrations and gingival recession, may be missed. It is, therefore, essential to give the soft tissues more than a cursory glance at examination, so that these

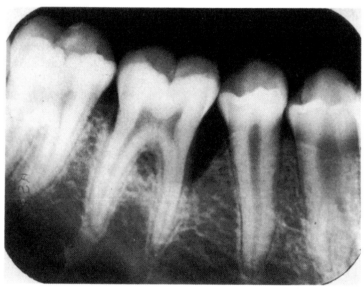

Fig. 2.2 *Periapical radiograph of the lower right posterior region of an 18-year-old boy, showing extensive bone loss around the first molar involving the furcation. This young man was unaware of any dental problems, and complained only of occasional bleeding on brushing when questioned. He has juvenile periodontitis.*

visible conditions may be detected early. Restorations should be examined carefully for overhanging margins, for they act as plaque traps and may compromise the periodontium.

JUVENILE PERIODONTITIS

This is the most common periodontal condition causing tooth loss in young people (over about 13 years). In Western Europe it occurs in 0.1% of children. Females are three times more likely to be affected than males, and there is a higher incidence in the negro population than among caucasians. In the classic form of juvenile periodontitis (also known as localised juvenile periodontitis) the first molars and maxillary incisors are affected. A more generalised form of the disease sometimes occurs, but rarely will the six index teeth used for screening not be involved.

The aetiology of juvenile periodontitis is not fully understood, but plaque levels tend to be low. Minor defects in host immunological mechanisms have been implicated, as have specific microorganisms in the plaque (e.g. *Actinobacillus actinomycetemcomitans*). Treatment (*see* Chapter 6, p. 43) includes deep scaling, root planing and oral hygiene instruction. Systemic antibiotic therapy in the active phases of the disease may be used. Oral hygiene instruction and frequent professional cleaning is often augmented with chlorhexidene gluconate mouthrinses.

REFERENCES

1. Matsson L., Golberg P. (1985). Gingival inflammatory reaction in children of different ages. *J. Clin. Periodontol*; **12**: 98–103.
2. Ainamo J., Barmes D., Beagrie G., *et al.* (1982). Development of the World Health Organization (WHO) Community Periodontal Index of Treatment Needs (CPITN). *Int. Dent. J*; **32**: 281–91.
3. Van Der Velden U., Winkel E. G., Abbas F. (1985). Bleeding/plaque ratio. A possible prognostic indicator of periodontal breakdown. *J. Clin. Periodontol*; **12**: 861–6.
4. Massler M., Schour I. (1949). The PMA index of gingivitis. *J. Dent. Res*; **28**: 634.
5. Ainamo J., Nordblad A., Kallio P. (1984). Use of the CPITN in populations under 20 years of age. *Int. Dent. J*; **34**: 285–91.
6. FDI. (1985). A simplified periodontal examination for dental practices. *Aust. Dent. J*; **30**: 368–70.

3

Current Understanding of the Caries Process

R. J. ELDERTON

For too long dental caries has been seen as a condition which, once started, progresses unhindered until a restoration is placed or the tooth is extracted. But this is far from the truth, since caries is a bacterial disease which is intermittent in nature. Its activity varies according to the level of activity of the bacteria involved.

The important essentials for caries are well known: a susceptible tooth, bacterial plaque and dietary sugar. While all of these are present to some extent in most mouths, the outcome of their interaction in terms of caries is entirely dependent upon the time factor. The frequency and duration of this interaction makes all the difference between the tooth surface remaining sound, a carious lesion developing, and a carious lesion arresting.

A DYNAMIC PROCESS

Dental caries is a dynamic process with periods of demineralisation and periods of remineralisation[1]. The enamel is normally in dynamic equilibrium with the saliva which, with respect to the enamel, is over-saturated with calcium and phosphate ions. However, in regions where there is bacterial plaque, dietary sugar is broken down by the enzymic processes of the plaque organisms to produce acid, and the pH falls. Once this begins to happen, the dental environment rapidly reaches a state of under-saturation with respect to calcium and phosphate ions, resulting in a tendency for these ions to diffuse out of the enamel. Demineralisation begins. Once the pH rises again, the saliva tries to give these ions back to the enamel (aided by fluoride where present) allowing the ionic balance to tip towards remineralisation. This oscillation of the balance and associated ionic exchange may occur many times each day as the oral environment changes in response to oral hygiene and dietary factors.

When the overall ionic balance at the enamel surface over a period of time is tipped towards demineralisation, the sides of the enamel prisms in the layer under the surface (the subsurface layer) are first dissolved away, leaving a relatively intact surface zone. As spaces develop between the prisms, so the region becomes more porous. A white spot carious lesion develops.

ENAMEL CARIES

The early carious lesion in enamel consists of four well-recognised histological zones. While two of these (the body of the lesion and the translucent zone) are produced by demineralisation, the other two are formed as a result of remineralisation[1].

The enamel crystals in the remineralising zones are significantly larger, at up to twice the diameter, than those of sound enamel. The new crystals thus have a more favourable surface area-to-volume ratio, a characteristic which will inevitably result in a reduction in their dissolution rate during any subsequent periods of potential demineralisation. Also, these newly-formed crystals contain significantly more fluoride than is found in adjacent sound enamel. The carious lesion, therefore, acts as a fluoride ion reservoir favouring remineralisation. The spaces created during demineralisation allow crystal growth to take place.

If overall demineralisation continues, complete breakdown of the enamel inevitably takes place, allowing a frank cavity to develop (Fig. 3.1, p. 16). However, if the conditions are altered so that the ionic balance is predominantly in the other direction, the overall effect will be remineralisation. Backer Dirks[2] and others have shown convincingly that early carious lesions can regress. Thus reversals in diagnosis have been reported whereby lesions detected clinically and by bitewing radiography had disappeared when examined at a later date using identical criteria.

As an individual gets older and the fluoride content of the surface enamel builds up from the various sources, so the chances of a carious lesion developing reduce automatically. It is indeed gratifying to realise that the ionic balance is always trying to move to the favourable side and this factor should not be ignored when

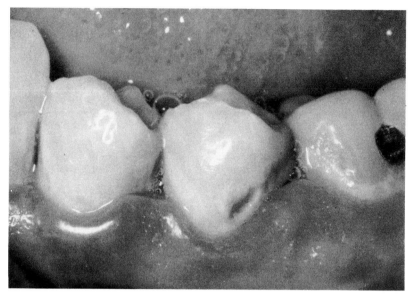

Fig. 3.1 *Lower posterior teeth in a 16-year-old girl who habitually chewed sugary gum. Considerable areas of demineralisation can be seen at the cervical margins of the teeth, cavitation finally taking place in the second premolar. Preventive management to bring about a change in the environment of these teeth provides the only hope of stopping the disease. Note the poor state of the gingival tissues.*

assessing the likelihood of a carious lesion in an individual being active, arrestable or arrested.

It will be appreciated that early caries in a pit or fissure often first manifests itself as white spot lesions in the sides of the fissure (*see* Plate 2), subsequently taking on a brown colour (*see* Plate 3) and spreading around the base of the fissure to become a single lesion (Fig. 3.2). Stages in the progression of the disease are the same as for smooth caries, though the invaginated morphology of the fissure has the effect of reducing the visible size of the lesion. An idea of the extent of the spread of the caries into the dentine can sometimes be determined from a bitewing radiograph (Fig. 3.3, p. 18).

DENTINE CARIES

The enamel surface is still intact when a carious lesion reaches the amelodentinal junction, and at this stage with an approximal

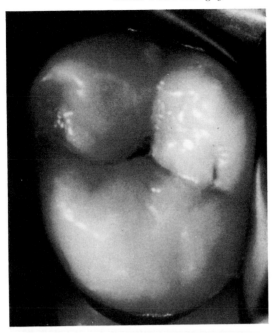

Fig. 3.2 *Upper molar with an occlusal carious lesion that has begun to under-mine the enamel, causing some breakdown to occur and a frank, darkly stained cavity to develop. The lesion may or may not be active, a matter which probing will not help to resolve.* (Reproduced by kind permission of A. E. Morgan, publishers of *Restorative Dentistry*.)

lesion, the tooth appears caries-free upon bitewing radiography. Once the enamel cavitates, bacteria are able to penetrate the tissue and the rate of progression of the lesion can be expected to increase, especially when the softer dentine is involved. However, progression usually remains remarkably slow, though surprisingly little is known of the natural history of caries and of the extent of variation in this natural history for different individuals and different communities. As with enamel caries, lesions in the dentine may become arrested and remain so (*see* Plate 4).

PROGRESSION OF CARIES

While caries may progress very fast in a few individuals, this is far from the norm. A review of 19 studies of the rate of progression of approximal caries determined from bitewing radiographs

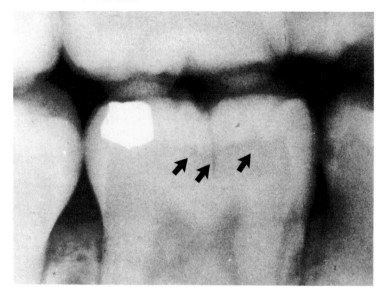

Fig. 3.3 *Part of a bitewing radiograph showing (arrows) early, but definite, spread of occlusal caries into the dentine. On histological examination, the lesion would be shown to have advanced further than the radiographic appearance suggests. The caries may or may not be active.*

revealed wide variation[3]. However, the general finding was that for most people, approximal caries progresses slowly, many lesions remaining unchanged for long periods. The mean time during which the lesions in this review remained confined radiographically to the enamel was 3–4 years. Backer Dirks[2], who examined children annually at ages 7–15 years with bitewing radiography, found that 50% of the lesions did not progress during 4 years, and that 26% remained unchanged over 8 years.

As with smooth surface lesions, early carious lesions in pits and fissures also may not progress. In four rather heterogeneous studies[4] of permanent molars in children, occlusal fissures that had been recorded as having early carious lesions were re-examined 24 to 41 months later, at which times 27% to 53% of the fissures were considered either to have reversed to a non-carious state or to have remained intact. Findings such as these should, of course, be balanced against the certain knowledge that high-risk individuals also exist in the community (*see* Chapter 4, p. 20), and that for these people, only a fastidious preventive programme is likely to meet with such success.

REFERENCES

1. Silverstone L. M. (1983). Remineralization and enamel caries: new concepts. *Dent. Update*; **10**: 261–73.
2. Backer Dirks O. (1966). Posteruptive changes in dental enamel. *J. Dent. Res*; **45**: 503–11.
3. Pitts N. B. (1983). Monitoring of caries progression in permanent and primary posterior approximal enamel by bitewing radiography. *Community Dent. Oral Epidemiol*; **11**: 228–35.
4. Elderton R. J. (1985). Management of early dental caries in fissures with fissure sealant. *Brit. Dent. J*; **158**: 254–8.

4

Assessment of Caries Risk and the Potential for Preventive Management

A. S. BLINKHORN and D. A. M. GEDDES

Good dental health is a valuable asset and an achievable goal for most patients. However, in spite of the general decline in the prevalence of dental caries in Western industrialised countries[1], improvements in dental health have not been universal and many children still suffer unacceptably high levels of the disease[2]. Fortunately, dentists can now spend more time on these individuals, and thus an immediate challenge for dentists in the field of caries prevention is to identify accurately those patients who are particularly at risk of developing carious lesions and to offer them appropriate care. There is no doubt at all that the probability of developing dental disease can be reduced if patients are helped to implement patterns of behaviour conducive to dental health. To do this, the dentist must learn enough about the patient to be able to tailor his advice appropriately and offer care which is relevant to the individual.

A detailed consultation and examination are crucial to the planning of a preventive programme geared to the needs of the patient at risk. The process of diagnosis and treatment planning can be optimised by utilising all the information available, so that as accurate an assessment as possible can be made of the risk factors and of their likely influence on future dental health.

The dentist responsible for the child should encourage in the parents the concept of oral health care. In this way, preventive advice can be given from birth. It is far more positive to *shape* behaviour rather than to change ingrained detrimental dental habits in the older child or adult.

THE CONSULTATION

The ability to elicit a full, accurate and relevant history from a patient is one of the most important skills for a dentist to develop; yet this aspect of dentistry has often received insufficient attention in undergraduate and postgraduate training. A comprehensive history enables the dentist to assess whether there are any physical, mental, medical or social problems which will enhance the susceptibility to dental disease or inhibit a patient's ability to comply with preventive treatment or advice that may be offered. Thus, there may be conditions whereby the biology of the oral cavity is altered on a regular basis. For example, children on regular antibiotic therapy administered in a sugary syrup will frequently have the ion exchange at the enamel/plaque interface shifted towards demineralisation, thereby enhancing the likelihood of caries development. Children who repeatedly consume sugary snacks and sweets throughout the day will also prejudice the ionic stability of the tooth enamel. Clearly, the identification of such information is an essential prerequisite for accurate caries prediction and prevention.

A social assessment will enable family attitudes to dental care to be determined. Usually, the district in which the family resides is closely related to social class, and evidence is available that the lower socio-economic groups do not have the same level of orientation to dental health as middle class families[3]. Once the clinician understands a patient's social circumstances, it is easier to establish a suitable programme of prevention. People in the lower social groups are also less likely to comprehend fully the technical terminology used by a health professional, this clearly restricting the level of communication that can be attained; words should be chosen that are appropriate to the knowledge and comprehension of the individual child and parent. The patient's previous dental experiences may provide clues as to the level of compliance that can be expected when offering advice on dental care.

Too often 'prevention' is not given the same priority by the dentist as clinical intervention. Thus, while dentists are usually good at predicting how long restorative procedures will take, they may not be good at gauging how long it is likely to take to bring about behaviour conducive to sound dental health. They may also be poor at making realistic assessments of how effective such conditioning is likely to be. Indeed, behavioural psychology is only now becoming an established part of dental education, so most dentists have received little training in helping patients to modify their behaviour.

Interviewing is a skill that is not readily acquired, and naivety in this area is highlighted by the number of health professionals who concentrate still on the 'why' approach to questioning. 'Why' is seen as potentially threatening by many people and, as a defence, responses are guarded. Specific questions the dentist should ask the parent or child depend very much on the individual, and on the individual's level of dental health. In order to gain a realistic insight into the way in which patients and their parents may respond to both preventive advice and treatment procedures, information is required on the individual's current level of knowledge and attitudes to dental care. Simplicity is a key to effective questioning, it being important to ask for information about only one thing at a time, and in a manner that is readily understood. Detailed questions will usually be required on the following topics:

- *Diet*—use a non-threatening approach and introduce the concept of a diet diary.
- *Oral hygiene*—although plaque and gingivitis can be measured, ascertain the patient's feelings about the value of oral hygiene.
- *Clinical care*—many parents place little value on the primary dentition, so it is important to assess, at a very early stage, any resistance to possible restorative components of a treatment plan for young children. Additional education may be an essential prerequisite to cooperation (and without this cooperation there may be little chance of dental health in adult life), and compromises in the treatment plan may be appropriate.
- *Transport*—too often treatment is planned without the dentist appreciating that travelling to the surgery may be difficult or that a parent may have a number of other young children to look after.

CLINICAL EXAMINATION

The clinical examination for the assessment of caries risk should form part of a careful review of the health of all the orofacial tissues. The amount of plaque present on the teeth provides an indication of the general level of dental self-care. However, as patients often clean their teeth just prior to a dental visit, the level of gingivitis may be a more reliable measure of toothbrushing. Small petechiae on the gingival tissue can reveal a patient's attempt to give the teeth a thorough previsit cleaning!

The presence or absence of teeth should be noted, for the early loss of primary or permanent teeth may give an indication of caries susceptibility. The teeth should be carefully examined for the presence of caries. Identification of areas of decalcification or shadowing beneath the enamel is best achieved by visual inspection under a bright light after all plaque has been removed and the teeth have been isolated with cotton wool rolls and dried in a stream of air. A probe should be used only as a cleaning tool during this examination, so as to avoid disrupting the tooth tissues and causing an open cavity in a decalcified area, thereby aiding the ingress of bacteria (*see* Chapter 11, p. 74).

DIAGNOSTIC AIDS

Radiography

One of the most important sources of information on which to base the diagnosis of dental caries is a radiographic examination. Every new patient should have bitewing radiographs taken to assess the extent of any posterior approximal or occlusal lesions. Radiographic assessment is particularly important in the primary dentition where the wide contact areas between the molars make visual examination very difficult.

The probability of the presence of an open cavity is low when a carious lesion is radiographically confined to the enamel. Indeed, most authorities agree that restorative intervention should not be undertaken for an approximal lesion unless it is radiographically through the amelodentinal junction (*see* Chapter 11, p. 75). Certainly, in an individual case, the decision as to whether or not to place a restoration for a small lesion should be made on more information than is provided by one radiograph; ideally, a series of radiographic findings obtained over a period of time should be considered together before making the decision.

It is important to minimise the frequency of exposure to radiation, which could otherwise be more than desirable in regular attenders with a low caries experience. As a general rule, patients who attend regularly for dental care should only be subjected to a radiographic examination at 2-yearly intervals. Patients with high caries rates may, however, in the first year or two of regular care, require radiographs taken more frequently in order to monitor the effects of preventive regimes.

Transillumination

Attempts have been made recently to refine caries diagnosis by the use of transillumination to highlight areas of demineralisation, and a fibre-optic light probe used for this purpose has been found to be a useful method for detecting early approximal lesions[4] in anterior teeth.

Electronic Caries Detection

A method of diagnosing caries by measuring electrical conductivity has also been proposed. The principle is that the conductivity of enamel varies according to the degree of mineral present, measurement being possible because microscopic porosities formed during demineralisation fill with saliva, providing highly conductive pathways for electrical transmission. The Vanguard caries detector (Massachusetts Manufacturing Corporation, Cambridge, Massachusetts, USA) is a portable battery operated device for this purpose, which is used to probe the occlusal surface of a tooth and produce a numerical conductivity reading. While further development of the instrument might lead to the production of a clinically reliable tool for occlusal caries assessment, *in vitro* studies have produced inconclusive results[5].

Diet Assessment

An important non-invasive aid for identifying individuals who are at high risk to caries is the diet diary (*see* Chapter 7, p. 47). Not only does this serve to pinpoint individuals who may need specific dietary advice, but it is a valuable tool in providing a basis for such advice.

Dietary education must be tempered by the fact that the confectionery companies spend large sums of money advertising the organoleptic pleasures of repeated consumption of sugary foods. Therefore, advice on reducing the consumption of sugary items should centre on regulating the specific times at which they are eaten, rather than attempting a complete change in dietary habits. Thus the major emphasis of dietary education should revolve around controlling the frequent consumption of potentially cariogenic items between meals. Modification of the diet through deletion of specific sugary foods/drinks, and their partial substitution with non-cariogenic items is the key to successful patient compliance.

Caries Activity Tests

Dental researchers are currently assessing various other objective ways of predicting the susceptibility to dental caries. Among these are 'Caries Activity Tests' (to use the generic term) which have included:

- *Lactobacillus* counts;
- assessments of *Streptococcus mutans* levels;
- saliva flow rates;
- saliva buffering capacity;
- determinations of the rate of sugar clearance from the oral cavity.

The usefulness of these tests as predictors of future caries in individual patients remains in doubt[6], though strong correlations have been found in epidemiological studies. If future research does validate the use of objective laboratory-based tests, this would be a significant breakthrough.

Caries activity tests are currently available commercially, e.g. the 'Dentocult–LB' (available from Rexodent Limited, 25–27 Merrick Road, Southall, Middlesex UB2 4AU). This is a simple dip-slide test for objective counting of salivary *Lactobacilli*. The patient stimulates salivation by chewing on a piece of paraffin wax, and expectorates into a paper cup. The dip-slide, which comes impregnated with rogosa sugar, is washed with the saliva and then incubated at 37°C for 4 days or at room temperature for 7 days. Interpretation of the cultured test is obtained by comparing the extent of the growth on the slide with those on a master printed card showing a range of characteristic growths.

Notwithstanding the fact that the validity of these tests for caries prediction in the individual patient is unproven, they can be used to motivate individuals to alter their oral flora by changing the intake of refined carbohydrates. The test can then be repeated to demonstrate the effect of the diet modification. Thus the use of saliva-related tests should be seen, at the present time, as a tool for motivation rather than for caries prediction.

INTERPRETATION OF THE DATA

Preventive and restorative treatment planning should be based on the collation of all the available information about the patient. Over-reliance on one source of information, such as radiographs, for implementing or witholding clinical intervention can result in both under- and over-treatment.

The scheme presented in Fig. 4.1 can be used to categorise patients into high or low caries risk groups. Once this information has been assimilated, an appropriate course of action can be drawn up. This may include elements of clinical preventive care to be initiated or provided by the dental team, and other specific action to be undertaken by the patients and/or parents. Taking all things into account, a realistic set of objectives can be presented to the individual. In order to avoid failure by being over ambitious, the good clinician will plan care in a realistic manner and not apply 'blunderbuss' preventive programmes in a standard 'take it or leave it' format.

The reader will appreciate that there is considerable evidence to show that the progress of early carious lesions through enamel is often slow and that many remain unchanged for long periods of time (*see* Chapters 3 and 11, pp. 14, 74), particularly in the permanent dentition, and that some lesions become arrested, especially if fluoride regimes are prescribed and appropriate dietary and oral hygiene changes are achieved. But as it is not necessarily possible to be sure which lesions will arrest, proper monitoring is essential.

This monitoring, together with criteria for treatment decision-making, must be adjusted according to the degree of success achieved with preventive measures. A variable recall system will be required. Reviews at 4-monthly intervals are recommended for very caries-prone individuals up until the time that the second

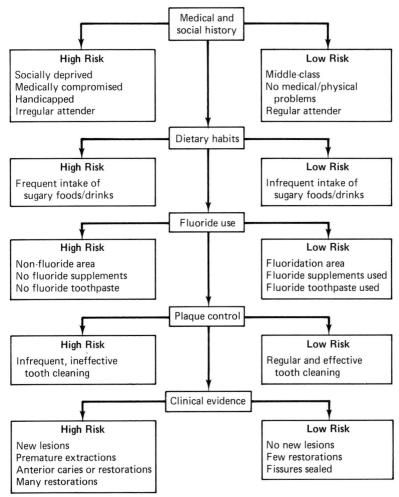

Fig. 4.1 *Flow diagram showing five types of data to be considered when assessing the caries risk of individual patients.*

permanent molars have been in the mouth for a year or two. After that time, or when the disease can be judged to be reasonably under control, 6-monthly examinations make sense for caries-prone individuals, but annual checks would seem appropriate for those with low caries experience[7]. A periodontal (*see* Chapters 2 and 6, pp. 7, 39) or other condition may, of course, dictate the need for more frequent visits. It will be appreciated, however, that while an annual screening may be sufficient *at the time* for a child with a sound dentition, this regime ignores the fact that the child's dental health status can change rapidly. The dentist has, therefore, to be continually on guard watching out for signs that dental care is slipping, and be prepared to take the necessary action, including reinforcing the preventive measures and increasing the recall frequency. From the behavioural point of view, it is important to encourage the habit of regular dental screening from an early age so that, subsequently as an adult, this pattern of attendance can be maintained as necessary.

REFERENCES

1. Downer M. C. (1984). Changing patterns of disease in the Western world. In: *Cariology Today*. (Guggenheim B., ed.). Basel: Karger.
2. Blinkhorn A. S., Cummins J., MacMillan A. S., O'Mailley G. (1985). Dental health of a sample of Glasgow adolescents. *Brit. Dent. J*; **158**: 436–9.
3. Blinkhorn A. S. (1981). Dental health education. In *An Introduction to Community Dental Health*. (Slack G. L., ed.). Bristol: John Wright and Sons.
4. Stephen K. W., Russell J. I., Creanor S. L., Burchell C. K. (1987). Comparison of fibre optic transillumination with clinical and radiographic caries diagnosis. *Community Dent. Oral Epidemiol*; **15**: 90–4.
5. Flaitz C. M., Hicks M. J., Silverstone L. M. (1986). Radiographic, histologic, and electronic comparison of occlusal caries: an in vitro study. *Pediatric Dent*; **8**: 24–8.
6. Bratthall D., Carlsson J. (1986). Current status of caries activity tests. In: *Textbook of Cariology*. (Thylstrup A., Fejerskov O., eds.). Copenhagen: Munksgaard.
7. Elderton R. J. (1985). Six-monthly examinations for dental caries. *Brit. Dent. J*; **158**: 370–4.

5

Early Detection of Malocclusion

I. D. BROWN

Any dentist who is caring for growing children should be looking out for occlusal abnormalities. By doing this, appropriate interceptive treatment can be given or the children referred for advice at the right time so that subsequent complicated treatment or the development of a handicapped dentition is avoided.

What are the factors responsible for the erupted positions of the teeth? It is generally agreed that the position of the apices of the teeth is determined by the basal bones of the jaws, whereas the position of the crowns is determined by the moulding influence of the lips and cheeks on the outside of the dental arches, and the tongue on the inside. If the combined mesio-distal widths of the teeth are greater than the dental arch length (a common finding in NW Europe) then the dentition will be crowded. These factors, i.e. the size, shape and relationship of the basal bones of the jaws and of the surrounding soft tissues are, together with tooth size, genetically determined. Thus, for example, the fact that a given child has a Class III malocclusion with crowding in both arches, would have been decided at the moment of conception.

REASONS FOR ELIMINATING MALOCCLUSIONS

The objectives of orthodontic treatment are frequently aesthetic; to give the dentition a pleasing appearance. There are, however, some relatively rare functional reasons for advising treatment. For example, a patient with a Class II malocclusion may have a potentially traumatic overbite which could eventually lead to periodontal damage and many years of annoying discomfort if left untreated. Also, a unilateral posterior crossbite may be associated with a deviation of the mandible towards the affected side on closure; this may lead to temporomandibular joint problems in later life if left untreated[1].

Parents often ask whether the presence of untreated crowding would increase the likelihood of caries and periodontal disease. Unfortunately, there is a little convincing evidence either way. A recent report on school children in England and Wales noted significantly more dental caries and gingival inflammation in children with crowded dentitions[2]. Dickson[3], however, investigated the long-term effects of malocclusion by comparing a group of dentate over 65-year-olds with younger age groups and concluded that loss of teeth, from whatever cause, is little affected by the degree of crowding.

If having well-aligned teeth results in the individuals concerned being more likely to take care of them and listen to advice, then orthodontic treatment in childhood may be expected to lead to a greater likelihood of dental health in adult life.

OCCLUSAL ASSESSMENT IN THE MIXED DENTITION

At 8 to 9 years of age following the eruption of the permanent incisors, it is possible to classify a patient's occlusion and obtain some indication of the severity of any crowding. Any space required for the alleviation of crowding or for overjet reduction will have to be provided for by the extraction of permanent teeth. First premolars are often the prime choice, as their extraction provides space close to where it is required. It follows, therefore, that orthodontic treatment for situations such as these cannot start until the maxillary canines and first premolars have erupted.

It is an old orthodontic adage that when considering the choice of extractions, the questions asked by the clinician should be: 'First premolars? If not, then why not?'. The reasons 'why not?' are usually because other permanent teeth are either of poor prognosis, have abnormal form, are grossly displaced or are missing. The dentist who looks after the patient has an ideal opportunity, and indeed an obligation, to make sure that the patient's dentition is developing normally and that any necessary remedial action is taken at the optimum time, and with specialist advice where appropriate.

The mixed dentition should not be looked upon as a period of inactivity while waiting until the deciduous teeth are shed.

Indeed, there are situations (*see* below and Chapter 14, p. 96) where, for example, the timely extraction of deciduous teeth can considerably simplify, and at times obviate, future orthodontic treatment.

DEVELOPMENTALLY ABSENT TEETH AND SUPER-NUMERARY TEETH

At 8 years of age all permanent teeth, apart from most third molars, should be present on radiographs. It is sound practice, therefore, to take orthopantomogram (OPG) (or left and right lateral obliques) and nasal occlusal radiographs at this age as a routine screening procedure in order to determine whether any permanent teeth mesial to the first permanent molars are developmentally absent and, unless experienced, to refer the patient for specialist advice if this is found to be so. The nasal occlusal radiograph is necessary because OPGs[4] and lateral oblique radiographs cannot be relied upon to give accurate representation of the anterior teeth. Where second premolars are developmentally absent and the incisors are crowded, extraction of the second deciduous molars (carried out early enough in the mixed dentition stage) can result in sufficient spontaneous alignment so that crowding is resolved and adequate space closure produced (Fig. 5.1*a* and *b*, p. 32).

The most common reason for the clinical absence of maxillary lateral incisors is agenesis, whereas when a maxillary central incisor fails to appear in the mouth, a supernumerary tooth is usually present preventing its eruption. Indeed, where one or both of the deciduous maxillary central incisors have been retained and yet the permanent lateral incisors have erupted, it should be assumed that a supernumerary tooth is responsible. This should be confirmed with a nasal occlusal radiograph. If found to be present, the supernumerary should be removed at an early stage while the unerupted incisor still has sufficient eruptive force to erupt spontaneously without recourse to exposure and traction. However, a full assessment should first be made, as teeth other than the supernumerary frequently need to be removed in addition. For example, if there is insufficient space to accommodate the unerupted incisor within the arch, then extraction of the two maxillary deciduous canines should also be carried out. Failure

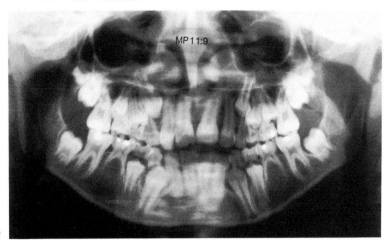

a

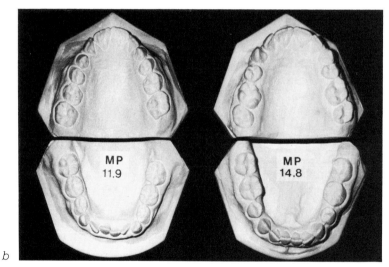

b

Fig. 5.1a and *b* *a = OPG of a patient aged 11 years and 9 months with a Class II division 1 malocclusion and lower arch crowding, but in whom the lower second premolars were developmentally absent. b = Occlusal view of the study models before and after orthodontic treatment. All the deciduous canines and molars were removed at 11 years and 9 months of age, followed by the upper second premolars when they had erupted. Upper removable appliances were used to retract the first premolars and upper canines, and then reduce the overjet. No appliances were used in the lower arch where space closure has been very good.*

to do so will often result in the permanent incisor remaining unerupted even though the blocking supernumerary has been removed.[5].

MISPLACED MAXILLARY CANINES

By the time the first premolars erupt, at about 10 years of age, the maxillary deciduous canines should be loosening and the unerupted maxillary permanent canines should be palpable as obvious bulges in the buccal sulci. Failure to elicit these signs could mean that the permanent canine in question is developing ectopically, it being rare for these teeth to be developmentally absent. Suspicion should be aroused whenever there is a retained but firm maxillary deciduous canine in one quadrant and yet the contralateral permanent canine has erupted; *always beware of asymmetry*. Radiographic investigation with parallax views (Fig. 5.2a, p. 34) is required in order to determine the position of the crown of the unerupted canine with respect to the root of the lateral incisor. The majority of misdirected maxillary canines are palatally placed and would eventually become noticeable as a bulging of the palatal mucoperiosteum. Others remain high and horizontal, the crowns lying buccal to the apex of the lateral incisor.

Misplaced maxillary canines can certainly be aligned by orthodontic means, but an early start is desirable. There is then a good chance that a palatally placed canine will improve spontaneously following the extraction of the deciduous canine and the provision of adequate space by orthodontic means[6] (Fig. 5.2a and b, p. 34). Orthodontic treatment in these situations is therefore relatively simple. However, if spontaneous improvement does not occur and surgical exposure *is* required, then by starting early, the patient would at least be more likely to go along with what would amount to being a fairly prolonged course (2–3 years) of treatment. If left to, say, 14 years of age or older, patients are not always committed enough to tolerate this treatment.

ANTERIOR CROSSBITES

One or more maxillary permanent incisors may erupt into crossbite. If at least one maxillary incisor is not in crossbite, then those

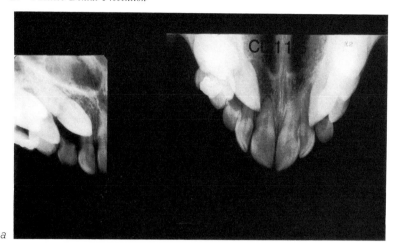

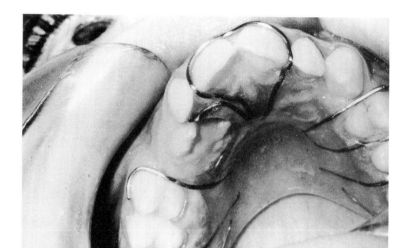

Fig. 5.2a and **b** a = *Periapical (left) and nasal occlusal radiographs (right) used to investigate the position of the unerupted upper right canine in a patient aged 11 years and 5 months. Using the principle of parallax, it can be seen that the canine is palatally placed with respect to the root of the lateral incisor. b = Following extraction of the deciduous canine and the use of an orthodontic appliance to move the right maxillary buccal segment distally, there has been spontaneous eruption of the canine. A retaining appliance is shown.*

incisors that are can be expected to be stable if moved labially to similar positions. Treatment for these patients can be considered during the mixed dentition (Fig. 5.3*a*, *b* and *c*, pp. 36, 37). Where there is crowding, space can be created by extracting the four deciduous canines. This action will transfer the crowding to the canine region, and it can be treated later following the eruption of the first premolars.

When all of the maxillary permanent incisors are in crossbite, specialist advice will be required at the mixed dentition stage. While some of these patients can be treated at that time with removable appliances, others are better treated in the permanent dentition with fixed appliances[7].

POSTERIOR CROSSBITES

Unilateral posterior crossbites associated with lateral deviation of the mandible to the affected side on closure should be treated by bilateral expansion of the maxillary dental arch. Most clinicians would choose to carry out this treatment in either the permanent or early mixed dentition so that there are no loose deciduous molars present to compromise appliance retention. An advantage of delaying treatment until the permanent dentition stage is that it is then possible to treat all aspects of the child's malocclusion during one phase of treatment.

Where there is a bilateral posterior crossbite or a unilateral posterior crossbite without deviation, the patient should be referred for specialist advice when the first premolars have erupted, in order to see whether it would be worthwhile correcting the crossbite as part of the patient's overall orthodontic treatment.

DIGIT SUCKING

Most children suck a digit at some time or other. The effect on the dentition depends upon the intensity and duration of the habit. Typically, it produces an anterior open bite and some increase in the overjet. The malformation produced is purely local in extent and restricted to the dento-alveolar structures, there being no alteration in the soft tissues and basal bones. Once the habit stops, the incisors show a strong tendency to erupt and align themselves. This is particularly true in the mixed dentition[8].

There is little point in fitting an appliance to break the habit in the deciduous and early mixed dentition. Indeed, it is desirable to leave children alone at this stage in view of the comfort that many of them obviously derive from the habit. An exception to this advice would be a child who has a unilateral posterior crossbite with lateral deviation on closure (commonly an associated finding with digit suckers) and who is keen to stop the habit. An appliance

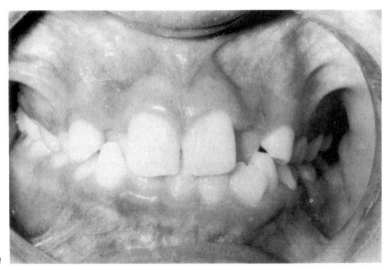

a

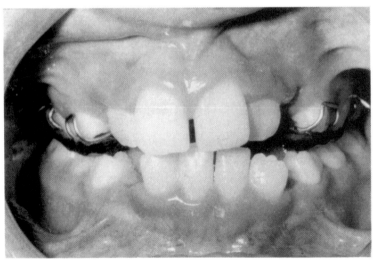

b

fitted to correct the crossbite in the early mixed dentition will also work to deter the habit.

If the habit persists when the first premolars and maxillary canines have erupted and active orthodontic treatment is to be undertaken (to reduce an overjet), the habit will often cease when the appliance is fitted. The open bite then often resolves spontaneously. However, anterior open bites maintained by digit sucking until the teenage years sometimes do not fully resolve even if the habit then ceases. In these cases, fixed appliances are necessary to extrude the maxillary incisors to the required level.

SUMMARY

1. Nasal occlusal and extra-oral radiographs (OPG or lateral obliques) should routinely be taken at 8 years of age in order to identify supernumerary teeth and/or developmentally absent permanent teeth.

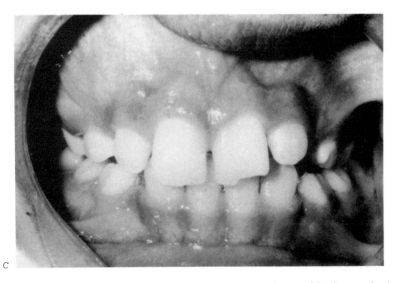

c

Fig. 5.3a, *b* and *c* *a = The maxillary lateral incisors in crossbite in a patient aged 9 years and 2 months. b = The four deciduous canines have been extracted to provide space for incisor alignment, and a removable appliance has been provided to move the lateral incisors labially. c = Three months later, the crossbite has been corrected. Unfortunately the incisal edge of the left central incisor was fractured during a fall.*

2. Digital palpation for unerupted maxillary permanent canines should routinely be carried out at 10 years of age. If there is then any doubt as to the position of these teeth, parallax radiographs should be taken.
3. Prompt referral for specialist advice is necessary for patients with abnormalities identified by these screening procedures in order to minimise the complexity of treatment.

REFERENCES

1. Egermark-Eriksson I., Ingervall B., Carlsson G. E. (1983). The dependence of mandibular dysfunction in children on functional and morphologic malocclusion. *Amer. J. Orthod*; **83**: 187–94.
2. Todd J. E. (1975). *Children's Dental Health in England and Wales, 1973.* pp. 70–3. London: HMSO.
3. Dickson G. C. (1974). Long term effects of malocclusion. *Brit. J. Orthod*; **1**: 63–8.
4. Rowse C. W. (1971). Notes on interpretation of the orthopantomogram. *Brit. Dent. J*; **131**: 425–34.
5. DiBiase D. D. (1971). The effects of variations in tooth morphology and position on eruption. *Dent. Practit*; **22**: 95–108.
6. Howard R. D. (1978). Impacted tooth position: unexpected improvements. *Brit. J. Orthod*; **5**: 87–92.
7. Mills J. R. E. (1982). Principles and practice of orthodontics. pp. 171–92. Edinburgh: Churchill Livingstone.
8. Bowden B. D. (1966). The effects of digital and dummy sucking on arch widths, overbite and overjet: A longitudinal study. *Aust. Dent. J*; **11**: 396–404.

6

Preventive Management of Periodontal Disease

J. LUKER

ORAL HYGIENE INSTRUCTION

Except where there is an underlying systemic predisposing condition, it is possible to prevent periodontal disease in informed subjects who are willing to participate in preventive care programmes. Even susceptible individuals with a defective host immune response to plaque (*see* Chapter 2, p. 7) can be free from disease, as they will not require a host response if the causative agent is removed.

Oral hygiene instruction should aim at achieving effective plaque removal and also at educating the individual so that the nature of periodontal disease is understood (*see* Plate 1). Of course, this is a goal which will only be achieved by those who are motivated and who are mentally and physically capable, but if oral hygiene instruction is begun in the young age groups, the individuals concerned will be conditioned to receiving and comprehending more advanced preventive material as they grow. Even though gingivitis is not common in the preschool child, oral hygiene should thus become part of the daily routine so that it becomes a habit. Though children under about 7 years of age do not have the manual dexterity to brush their teeth effectively, they should, nevertheless, be encouraged to brush for themselves so that it becomes a habit which may be expected to improve in quality by the time they *are* aged about 7 years, when, otherwise, the inflammatory reaction to plaque might begin to affect the periodontal tissues more earnestly. By using a fluoride toothpaste at the same time, these young children will also be availing themselves of an effective anti-caries measure.

Parental brushing is important for mentally handicapped children who will never have enough manual dexterity or understanding to brush effectively themselves. If this is carried out from an early age, it becomes incorporated into a regular daily routine which will probably have to be continued throughout life.

Children's toothbrushes should have small heads and soft bristles. It is not important which technique a child uses, providing it is effective for removing plaque; a general rotary scrubbing method is the easiest to teach, not forgetting to make the point that the bristles should, purposely, be angled towards the gingival margins, and that the gingiva itself should be the main target of the brush. It is also necessary to stress the importance of reaching all areas of the mouth. Often it is more effective to modify a child's existing technique than to teach a new one. Plaque can easily be demonstrated to the child with disclosing tablets or solution, which can be used both at home and in the surgery.

The use of dental floss cannot be mastered until a child has developed a high level of manual dexterity. This eliminates flossing as a realistic possibility for those under 12 years old who may, in any case, do more harm than good with floss if they try it.

Flossing can best be taught directly in the mouth so that the child can be shown precisely how to hold it and angle it between the teeth. The gentle insertion of floss and its gradual easing past the contact points until it rests on the gingival crevice should be practised by the child under supervision. Its action can be explained by showing that with gentle pressure against the tooth, the floss fibres will splay out to disturb and trap the plaque, and then hold it as the floss is drawn along the side of the tooth. Incorrect ways of using floss can also be demonstrated, such as sawing actions which may cut the gingiva. It is realistic for the child to begin flossing only on the anterior teeth; once this has been mastered, he or she can progress to the more difficult posterior teeth.

A school child is often very much under parental control, and parents who are not themselves concerned with oral hygiene may not help in instilling oral hygiene habits in their children. It behoves the dentist to try to involve, educate and enthuse the parents as much as possible in an effort to enlist their encouragement for the child. With the handicapped, it is necessary to spend time instructing the parents or other helpers in oral hygiene regimes. It is often appreciated by all concerned if the instruction is of a practical type, with the patient and/or parent being advised on the basis of actually demonstrating the oral hygiene procedure in the patient's mouth. Switching to an electric brush may provide enormous uplift under these circumstances.

Where the necessary motivation and home care is lacking, regular professional cleaning may be appropriate. Though rather empirical, daily self-application of 0.4% stannous fluoride gel in custom made trays may have a role in the control of periodontal disease in these patients (and caries also). Less severely handicapped individuals may derive benefit from modified toothbrushes with enlarged, elongated or angled handles which make them easier to hold and manipulate. Group teaching is not effective for the handicapped, as individual needs may vary greatly. Each person requires assessment and a personalised oral health care programme.

Incompetent Lips and Mouthbreathing

Gingival hyperplasia associated with incompetent lips and mouthbreathing requires no special periodontal treatment unless there is evidence of bleeding on probing. Clearly any calculus deposits should be removed. If gingivectomy is undertaken to achieve an aesthetic improvement, it is important to wait for the correction, where possible, of any predisposing cause prior to treatment. If antiepileptic drugs are causing gingival hyperplasia, it may be realistic to consult the physician to see if the drug can be changed. Where this is not possible, frequent professional oral hygiene (ideally every 2 days, but more realistically once per month) may be required if the patient cannot maintain effective plaque control[1]. This also applies to hereditary gingivofibromatosis.

The occlusion should be checked, but orthodontic treatment as a periodontal measure is required only when there is direct trauma to the gingival margin (*see* Chapter 15, p. 119). While irregularities in tooth arrangement may predispose to plaque accumulation and benefit from orthodontic intervention, if plaque removal is effective, they should not exacerbate periodontal disease. A more certain way of aggravating periodontal disease would be to place an orthodontic appliance in the mouth of a child with ineffective plaque control.

SCALING

Perfect brushing and flossing is completely effective at plaque removal and therefore at preventing calculus formation. As this high standard is rarely maintained and plaque deposits are left which later calcify to form calculus, especially lingual to the mandibular incisors and molars and buccal to the maxillary molars, it is inevitable that scaling will be necessary in some patients. It should be emphasised that it is essential to remove (with a hand or ultrasonic scaler) the most apically positioned calculus, not because it causes direct trauma to the gingiva, but because it is always associated with bacterial plaque.

CHEMICAL CONTROL OF PLAQUE

Chemical control of bacterial plaque is a useful adjunct to mechanical plaque removal, even in those receiving regular prophylaxis. Chlorhexidene gluconate as a 0.2% mouthwash used twice daily for periods up to 6–8 weeks has been shown to effectively reduce plaque and gingivitis even in mentally handicapped children. It should be rinsed around the mouth for 1–2 min once in the morning after brushing and once in the evening. If this mouthwash is unacceptable or if the patient is too young or uncooperative, a 1% oral chlorhexidine gel can be applied directly to the gingiva with a toothbrush. Side-effects include discoloration of the teeth and tongue and, very occasionally, parotid swelling. Unfortunately, both these chlorhexidine preparations have an unfavourable taste which, especially for children, may negate their acceptance. In this case, a proprietary preparation called Eludril, which contains a lower concentration of chlorhexidine combined with other antiseptics, is available as an alternative in the form of a pleasant, cherry-flavoured mouthwash or spray.

The 0.2% chlorhexidine mouthwash should be used by the dentist as frequently as possible to irrigate active pathological pockets during active phases of periodontal disease as, for example, in juvenile periodontitis. The solution is drawn into a 2 ml sterile hypodermic syringe with a blunted narrow gauge needle which is inserted carefully into the pocket. Gentle pressure is applied to the syringe until chlorhexidine flows from the pocket margin.

ANTIBIOTIC THERAPY

Systemic antibiotic therapy is only used in acute periodontal infections, such as acute necrotising ulcerative gingivitis (ANUG), periodontal abcesses (when drainage cannot be established and/or where there is cervical lymphadenopathy) and in advanced cases of periodontitis, such as (during active phases of) juvenile periodontitis.

ANUG may occur in children with leukaemia or in those with an immunological deficiency or other compromising medical condition. The antibiotic of choice for primary treatment of this condition is metronidazole 200 mg three times a day for adults and children over 12 years. For younger children the dose is approximately half, the precise dose being calculated according to body weight. Metronidazole is a specific antimicrobial agent against Gram-negative anaerobes. It is unlikely to cause an imbalance in the normal oral flora.

Tetracycline, a broad spectrum antibiotic, has been used with some success in the active phase of juvenile periodontitis. It also has a role prior to and after periodontal surgery. Tetracycline is not recommended in the Dental Practitioners' Formulary for use in children under 12 years of age; certainly unsightly incorporation of tetracycline into developing teeth (apart from the wisdom teeth) will not effect aesthetics if used at this age, the crowns of even the second molars usually having formed by the age of 8.

CHILDREN WITH ADVANCED PERIODONTAL DISEASE

It is rare to see advanced periodontal disease in a child under 16 years of age. If you do, think *why*? Advanced periodontal disease in this age group is usually a manifestation of an underlying systemic disorder (or juvenile periodontitis) which may affect the balance between host resistance and bacterial plaque, e.g. diabetes mellitis, leukaemia, aplastic anaemia or cyclic neutopenia.

It is advisable in these more complex cases to follow a treatment plan devised by a specialist in periodontology[2]. If it is not possible for the patient to attend in person (e.g. because of the distance involved), a consultant may be contacted for advice over the telephone or case notes and radiographs may be sent in an endeavour to obtain a written treatment plan. An example of such a treatment plan (though clearly, many variations are possible) might be as follows for a patient with juvenile periodontitis (*see* Fig. 2.2, p. 12):

Sample Treatment Plan for Juvenile Periodontitis

1. Thorough scaling, root planing and oral hygiene reinforcement. (Most patients with juvenile periodontitis have good oral hygiene.)
2. Irrigation of pockets which bleed on probing with 0.2% chlorhexidine gluconate.
3. Course of systemic antimicrobial therapy: tetracycline 250 mg q.d.s. for 2–3 weeks. (Often systemic antimicrobial agents deactivate pockets by changing their bacterial flora.)
4. After systemic antimicrobial therapy, reassess the activity of the disease:
   (a) if inactive, i.e. no bleeding on probing, go to step 9;
   (b) if some or all of the pockets bleed, arrange surgery.
5. Surgery to one quadrant, i.e. open curettage to remove any necrotic cementum, calculus and granulation tissues. (The surgical technique will vary between individual patients, but it generally requires an inverse bevel incision, removal of the epithelium lining the pocket, and replacement of the flap either in the original position or apically.)
6. During the initial postsurgical period, prescribe chlorhexidine gluconate 0.2% mouthwash b.d.s. for 2 weeks or until normal toothbrushing is resumed.
7. One week after the surgery, remove the sutures. Gently remove any plaque deposits surrounding the gingival margin of the treated area. Reinstitute gentle toothbrushing.
8. Reassess 1 month after the surgery:
   (a) If the treated area is quiescent, arrange surgery to the other active quadrants over the next 6 months.
   (b) If the treated area does not appear to have responded to the surgery, the prognosis is poor—return to step 1 of the treatment plan.
9. Following successful antimicrobial therapy at step 4, or after the surgery has been completed and the pockets are quiescent, reassess 3–4 monthly (if active pockets are identified, return to step 1) and then 6 monthly.

GENERAL

Prevention of periodontal diseases and their consequences are, without doubt, the best treatment for all children including the medically compromised, for this will give them the greatest chance of maintaining a healthy periodontium into adult life.

REFERENCES

1. Badersten A., Edelberg J., Koch G. (1975). Effect of monthly prophylaxis on caries and gingivitis in schoolchildren. *Community Dent. Oral Epidemiol*; **3**: 1–4.
2. Davies R. M. (1988). Periodontal diseases. In *The Dentition in Health and Disease*. (Elderton R. J., ed.). London: William Heinemann Medical Books. (In press.)

7

Diet Counselling and Oral Hygiene in Caries Control

J. J. MURRAY

To many people the idea of diet counselling is a rather tired message and it is easy for dentists to approach the subject half-heartedly, assuming they are going to have little chance of changing their patients' eating habits. But it is dietary items upon which dental plaque bacteria feed, and moderate or extensive levels of caries can usually be related to an inappropriate dietary pattern—one involving frequent or prolonged intakes of items containing sugar (with multiple or prolonged periods of potential demineralisation, and a relatively small amount of remineralisation time).

EXTENSIVE CARIES IN INFANTS

In very young children, 'dummy caries' is still a distinct clinical problem which causes much pain and suffering to the affected child, but which is totally preventable (*see* Plate 5). It is characterised by multiple labial lesions on the upper deciduous incisors, often associated with an anterior open bite. Canines and molars are often also affected. In most cases, the condition can be linked either to putting sugar or a sugary juice in the bottle, or coating a dummy with a sugary substance. New parents should be warned of these dangers (perhaps at the time they, themselves, present for dental care) so that they do not allow the habit to start.

Once started, the habit should, of course, be discontinued, and an effective way to do so is through a weaning process whereby the offending agent is gradually diluted with water until, eventually, plain water can be substituted and the habit dropped. Clearly, doctors, midwives and health visitors should be discouraged from recommending the addition of sugar to bottles or other foods, and sugar-free medicines should be normal practice for infants (indeed anyone) on long-term medication.

EXTENSIVE CARIES IN THE MIXED OR PERMANENT DENTITION

In spite of the recent decline in the disease, extensive caries is still found in the deciduous dentition in a proportion of young children, and early serious involvement of the first permanent molars is a force to be reckoned with. In many cases, a link with frequent sugar consumption can be ascertained.

Children and young people in the UK consume a very high proportion of all soft drinks[1]. Indeed, a recent study showed that 42% of squashes were consumed by children aged between 2 and 9 years, 23% by those aged between 10 and 15 years, 16% by young adults aged between 16 and 24 years, and only 19% by adults over 24 years. Further, it was noted that confectionery contributes 28% to the total amount of added sugar to the diet of teenage children. In a 2 year longitudinal study to determine the relationship between dietary habits and caries incidence in English adolescent school children, it was shown that those who consumed the most sugar (an average of 163 g a day) developed a mean DMFS of 5.0 during the 2 years, 56% more than the children who had the lowest sugar intake, a mean of 78 g a day.

DIET COUNSELLING

In patients with active caries, it is necessary to discuss with the child and parents in some detail the pattern of food and drink consumption. Diet counselling should be approached gently, with a view to trying to show the high frequency of sugar consumption, paying particular emphasis to any added and hidden sugar content of the diet. Doing this in a condemnatory tone is unlikely to achieve the desired effect. Parents often fail to appreciate that adding sugar to tea or coffee, or the frequent provision of dilute fruit juice drinks can have a profound effect on the number of times sugar is taken into the mouth each day.

One of the best ways to determine dietary information is to ask the parent (usually the mother) to fill in a 3-day diet history sheet. The days chosen should be a Thursday, Friday and Saturday, or a Sunday, Monday and Tuesday, so that one of the days surveyed falls on a weekend (and also represents the school holidays periods). Ask the mother to write down everything the child has to eat or drink, including snacks, and also to estimate quantities in terms of a bowlful, a spoonful, a cupful, etc. This latter information is helpful to the clinician when giving advice.

The diet sheet is then used to tailor a dietary discussion to the individual, with the specific aim of determining the number and frequency of items containing sugar, and then causing a reduction in these to, ideally, mealtimes only. In practical terms this is usually impossible, because old habits die hard and the child does not want to be seen to be deviating markedly from the habits of his or her peers. It should also be appreciated that alternative snack foods which do not contain sugar, are usually more expensive. Nevertheless, marked changes in dietary habits *can* realistically be brought about if the clinician is sufficiently enthusiastic and is able to impart an awareness that appropriate dietary changes are *essential* if the child is ever to reach maturity with a sound dentition which he or she can reasonably expect to keep healthy into adult life. Adolescents usually have a certain amount of financial independence, sometimes through money earned from paper rounds, and the newspaper shop that supplies the money also displays and sells canned drinks and a multitude of other tempting sugar-containing snacks. It is important to try to understand all these driving forces and to appreciate them in discussion with the patient. Specific suggestions include:

- give up sugar-containing boiled sweets that are packeted for isolated (frequent) consumption, and substitute 'all in one go' chocolate bars (which are more 'filling') and which do not, in the same way, add hugely to the daily number of intakes.
- restrict confectionery consumption to meal times;
- if sugar is placed in tea or coffee, substitute an artificial sweetener;
- if fruit drinks and squashes are consumed, substitute sugar-free varieties;
- if fizzy drinks are frequently mentioned, suggest 'diet' versions;

- try to replace some of the sweet snacks by fruit, crisps, nuts or cheese;
- try to limit sugar in both food and drinks to meal times only;
- never allow a sugar-containing drink to be consumed last thing at night.

THE ROLE OF ORAL HYGIENE

The role of oral hygiene in caries prevention and control is quite clear; the Health Education Council summed it up as 'clean the teeth and gums thoroughly every day with a fluoride toothpaste'. However, research findings have sometimes confused the message. Many studies have found a poor correlation between the prevalence of dental caries and the standard of oral hygiene, because the indices for measuring the caries (dmf, DMF) have been concerned with the accumulation of past disease and treatment, whereas the oral hygiene indices have attempted to assess the amount of plaque present on a given day at the time of the study.

Even in clinical trials, where successive estimations of oral cleanliness have been related to the increase in caries that has occurred over the same period, findings have not necessarily been clearcut. In a 3-year clinical trial of children initially aged 11–12 years, the caries increments of 42 children who had good oral cleanliness at annual examinations were compared with those of 106 children with poor oral cleanliness[2]. Those with clean teeth at each examination had the smallest mean increment of caries, but the difference was rather less than 0.5 DMFT and was not statistically significant. In a somewhat similar analysis, 59 children with consistently clean mouths had a mean increment of 7.6 DMFS over 3 years compared with a mean of 10.3 DMFS in 101 children with consistently dirty mouths, a difference which was statistically significant ($p < 0.05$)[3].

Prospective studies involving supervised plaque removal, with or without professional tooth cleaning, might be expected to show a clear relationship between plaque levels and caries incidence. Most of the studies on such school-based plaque control programmes have taken place in Scandinavia or North America. Broadly, the American studies have indicated that supervised daily disclosing, brushing and flossing in school has no obvious effect on caries, whereas the Scandinavian regime, based on regular professional prophylaxes, has been shown to be beneficial[4].

A 3-year professional plaque control programme for adolescents within the Community Dental Service in England provided a statistically insignificant result[5]. While the participants in the test group had better oral hygiene and less gingival bleeding at the end of the study than those in the control group, there were only slightly fewer new carious lesions in the test group, a mean DMFS increment of 2.7, compared with 3.4 in the control group. It was concluded that in the field conditions of this study, professional plaque control did not significantly reduce caries.

Naylor[6] summed up the situation by concluding that 'whilst it is true that without plaque there will be no caries, there is no consistent evidence that plaque control, at the standard generally practised, reduces caries experience; nor is there sufficient evidence to dismiss good oral cleanliness as a caries-preventive procedure'. But plaque control is of proven benefit in the prevention and treatment of periodontal disease, and anecdotal evidence witnessed by every dentist in the land supports the old adage that a clean tooth never decays.

FREQUENCY OF TOOTHBRUSHING

It is dangerous to equate *frequency* of toothbrushing with *effective* toothbrushing. The findings of the part of the 1973 survey, in which toothbrushing habits were related to tooth decay in 5-year-olds, showed very little difference between the groups. Indeed, the proportion caries-free in the category which brushed three times a day was 1% higher than among those who brushed less than once a day. Notwithstanding this, one look at any of the myriad of toothpaste trials that have been conducted over the past 40 years will surely convince anyone that regular brushing with a well formulated fluoride-containing toothpaste will help to reduce dental caries.

In practical terms, brushing every day makes good sense, and fewer thorough brushings are better than more frequent cursory brushings. However, a sense of realism should prevail, and it is important to appreciate the two different purposes of toothbrushing:

- to remove plaque;
- to apply a preventive/therapeutic dose of fluoride topically to the teeth.

Twice-daily brushing with fluoride toothpaste would seem to be appropriate advice for most people. Last thing at night is usually an acceptable time, and this has the benefit of supplying traces of fluoride for the long night of potential remineralisation time. After breakfast (or the hurried snack) is the other very practical time of the day to establish the routine. A sensible scrub technique should be advised, making sure that the toothbrush size and design allow the user to reach all tooth surfaces and gum margins.

REFERENCES

1. Rugg-Gunn A. J., Lennon M. A., Brown J. G. (1986). Sugar consumption in the United Kingdom. *Brit. Dent. J*; **161**: 359–64.
2. Sutcliffe P. (1973). A longitudinal clinical study of oral cleanliness and dental caries in school children. *Archs. Oral Biol*; **18**: 765–70.
3. Beal J. F., James P. M. C., Bradnock G., Anderson R. J. (1979). The relationship between dental cleanliness, dental caries incidence and gingival health. *Brit. Dent. J*; **146**: 111–14.
4. Ashley F. P., Sainsbury R. H. (1981). The effect of a school based plaque control programme on caries and gingivitis. A 3-year study in 11–14 year old girls. *Brit. Dent. J*; **150**: 41–5.
5. King J. M., Hardie J. M., Duckworth R. (1985). Dental caries and periodontal health following a professionally administered plaque control programme in adolescents. *Brit. Dent. J*; **158**: 52–4.
6. Naylor M. N. (1985). Possible factors underlying the decline in caries prevalence. *J. Roy. Soc. Med*; **78** (Suppl. 7): 23–5.

8

Fluorides and Caries

R. J. ANDLAW

FLUORIDATION TODAY

The benefits of water fluoridation in reducing the prevalence of dental caries have been noted in many parts of the world, from Grand Rapids in the USA which, in 1945, became the first city to fluoridate its water supply, to Birmingham and Newcastle in the UK, which introduced fluoridation in 1964 and 1968 respectively. However, while over 100 million people in the USA (about 60% of the population) drink fluoridated water, only about 3 million (about 6% of the population) do so in the UK. Though acknowledged as safe, wider implementation of fluoridation in the UK has been held up by political arguments and legal difficulties[1].

It is ironic that the passing of the Water (Fluoridation) Act in London in 1985, which removed legal barriers to the implementation of fluoridation, has coincided with a time of greatly reduced dental caries prevalence in the UK. Because of this caries reduction, the justification for introducing new fluoridation schemes in the UK now is often questioned. However, the improvement in dental health that has occurred has not been evenly distributed around the country and there are areas, especially in Scotland and the north of England (as well as in many other countries) where caries prevalence is still high; it would seem right to press for adjustment of the water supplies to an optimum fluoride level for all communities (where possible) in which the mean DMF at 12 years of age is greater than the World Health Organization goal of three.

OTHER METHODS OF USING FLUORIDE

In areas where the water supply contains little or no fluoride, the administration to children of a systematic fluoride supplement in the form of drops or tablets can confer protection against dental caries similar to that associated with the consumption of fluoridated water[2]. There is, however, the serious problem of motivating parents to continue giving these agents for the required number of years. This method of using fluoride must, therefore, be classed as a poor public health measure, for it is only likely to benefit those who are highly motivated—those who need it least. Fluoride tablets have been administered effectively in school programmes[3], but this requires the interest and cooperation of school staff, and children are only at school for about 200 days in the year.

By far the most important topical method is the home use of fluoride toothpaste (800–1500 ppm), but it should not be forgotten that fluoride mouthrinses (230 ppm for daily use; 900 ppm for weekly use) are also available for the patient to administer. Other topical methods include the professional application of a fluoride solution or gel (12 300 ppm) or varnish (23 000 ppm)[4], all of which have been shown to be effective.

RATIONALE FOR THE USE OF FLUORIDE SUPPLEMENTS AND TOPICAL FLUORIDE AGENTS

Current understanding of the use of fluorides has been documented recently by Murray[5].

Once or twice daily use of fluoride toothpaste is recommended for all dentate individuals. It is suggested that the decision as to whether or not to prescribe systemic fluoride supplements or to use additional topical fluoride methods should be based upon the assessment of two main risk factors: first, the predicted susceptibility of the individual to dental caries (*see* Chapter 4, p. 20), and secondly, the likelihood of general complications that would be associated with dental disease or dental treatment. Factors that should be considered include the following:

- clinical signs of high caries activity;
- high caries experience of older siblings of a young child;

- medical conditions that would be complicated by bacter-aemia resulting from infection or from some forms of dental treatment, e.g. congenital heart defects, or a history of rheumatic fever;
- medical conditions that make certain forms of dental treat-ment hazardous, e.g. a bleeding disorder;
- medical conditions which compromise the ability of body tissues to resist infection, e.g. diabetes, leukaemia;
- mental subnormality or physical handicap which makes dental treatment more than usually difficult to perform.

'High Risk' Child

If, after considering the factors outlined above, the child is clas-sified as 'high risk', systemic fluoride supplementation should be strongly encouraged if the patient lives in a low water-fluoride area. Administration may be commenced as early as is convenient to the parents, or it may be delayed until the baby is about 6 months old. The most convenient way to administer fluoride to an infant is to use drops, which may be added to a drink. Tablets should be used instead of drops as soon as the child is old enough to chew them, in order to gain the increased benefit of a topical as well as a systemic effect.

The recommended dosages for fluoride supplementation are given in Table 8.1[6]. Administration should continue at least until the age of 7 years, during which time the primary objective is to enhance fluoride uptake into the developing tooth structure. By maintaining the supplements until the premolars and second molars erupt there will be an additional advantage, as these teeth are still able to take up fluoride from the tissue fluid during their pre-eruptive maturation phase.

Especially for children with moderate amounts of active smooth

Table 8.1 *Recommended dosage of fluoride drops or tablets (mg F/day) related to the concentration of fluoride in the drinking water.*

Age (y)	Water F (ppm)		
	<0.3	0.3–0.7	>0.7
<2	0.25	0	0
2–4	0.50	0.25	0
>4	1.0	0.5	0

surface caries, topical methods are recommended in addition to systemic supplementation, even when fluoride toothpaste is being used. For children below the age of 5–6 years, the application of fluoride varnish is probably the most convenient method to use. For older children, the use of gel in a tray is often preferred. Applications should be carried out at least once a year, though preferably two or three times a year.

Children over the age of 7–8 years may be able to use a fluoride mouthrinse regularly at home to take the place of topical treatments in the surgery. Mouthrinsing should continue for several years after the premolars and second molars erupt, or longer if there is evidence of continued caries activity or if third molars are to take their places as useful members of the dentition.

Child not Classified as 'High Risk'

For children not classified as high risk, systemic fluoride supplements or surgery-based topical treatments are not routinely recommended, irrespective of the fluoride level in the water supply. This advice assumes, of course, that fluoride toothpaste is used regularly at home and that reasonable attention is being paid to maintaining good diet and oral hygiene habits. However, if the parents in a low fluoride area are highly motivated and keen to do everything possible to safeguard against caries, they may be informed of the possible benefits of using drops, tablets or rinses, though it is wise to counsel them carefully so that an excessive intake of fluoride is avoided. It cannot be denied that some additional anti-caries benefit could accrue from their use.

ENAMEL FLUOROSIS (MOTTLING)

The dosages given in Table 8.1 were published in 1981 after the matter had been reviewed by a working party of the British Dental Association. In agreement with recommendations made by the American Academy of Pediatrics and by the American Dental Association, the dose for children under the age of 4 years is lower than that previously accepted. Surveys have shown that a significant proportion of children receiving higher levels of fluoride supplementation had some degree of enamel fluorosis[7]. It is well known that cases of fluorosis have been noted among the children of dentists. It is expected that mottling will not occur with the lower dosages now recommended.

Another factor possibly associated with enamel fluorosis is the ingestion of fluoride toothpaste. Young children do not rinse or expectorate efficiently after toothbrushing and therefore they ingest some toothpaste. Studies have shown that the great majority of young children ingest less than 0.25 g of toothpaste (0.25 mg fluoride), but the occasional child may ingest as much as 1 g of paste (1 mg fluoride)[8]. There is no evidence that ingestion fluoride toothpaste *per se* causes mottling, but excessive ingestion of toothpaste is clearly undesirable for children already receiving systemic fluoride. Parents should be advised to supervise tooth-brushing by children and to limit the amount of toothpaste placed on the brush to about the size of a small pea.

REFERENCES

1. McKechnie R. (1985). The Strathclyde fluoridation case. *Community Dent. Hlth. 1985*; **2**: 63–8.
2. Forrester D. J., Schultz E. H., eds. (1974). International workshop on fluorides and dental caries reductions. p. 99. Baltimore: University of Maryland.
3. Stephen K. W. (1978). Caries reduction and cost benefit after 3 years of sucking fluoride tablets daily at school. *Brit. Dent. J*; **144**: 202–6.
4. Ripa L. W. (1981). Professionally (operator) applied topical fluoride therapy: a critique. *Int. Dent. J*; **31**: 105–20.
5. Murray J. J. (1986). Appropriate use of fluorides for human health. Geneva: FDI, W. K. Kellogg Foundation and World Health Organization.
6. Dowell T. B., Joyston-Bechal S. (1981). Fluoride supplements: age-related doses. *Brit. Dent. J*; **150**: 273–5.
7. Aasenden R., Peebles T. C. (1974). Effects of fluoride supplementation from birth on human deciduous and permanent teeth. *Arch. Oral Biol*; **19**: 321–6.
8. Hargreaves J. A., Ingram G. S., Wagg B. J. (1972). A gravimetric study of the ingestion of toothpaste by children. *Caries Res*; **6**: 237–43.

9

Problems with Restorative Dentistry

R. J. ELDERTON

In spite of preventive dentistry and the arresting of some carious lesions, the need for restorations will remain for the foreseeable future. However, restorative dentistry has occupied a central place in dentistry in the UK and in other parts of the developed world for so long that there has been considerable lethargy with respect to facing up to its shortcomings, and in keeping up-to-date with current concepts of cavity design and the use of restorative materials. One very serious result of this is that many patients have been handicapped for life as a result of inappropriate restorative treatment which sets their teeth at a restorative disadvantage—in that a repeat restoration cycle so easily becomes established. The corner has, however, been turned, and it is now clear that dentists are acknowledging many of the drawbacks of yesterday's restorative philosophy and are adopting a more cautious approach when deciding whether or not to restore or rerestore; and when they do restore, they are being more conservative in their cavity preparations.

In a text on prevention in childhood of dental disease in adult life, it is necessary to consider four clearly defined issues:

- shortcomings of outdated restorative treatment decisions (p. 58);
- shortcomings of outdated restorations and restorative procedures (*see* Chapter 10, p. 65);
- current concepts in the preventive management of dental caries (*see* Chapter 11, p. 74);
- current concepts of preventively-orientated restorations and restorative procedures (*see* Chapter 12, p. 82).

SHORTCOMINGS OF OUTDATED RESTORATIVE TREATMENT DECISIONS

Restorations do not Cure Caries

Restorative dentistry is based upon the concept that the surgical excision of carious tissue followed by restoration of the tooth is the treatment of choice for caries. With the possible exception of certain uses of glass-ionomer cement, these procedures in themselves, of course, do not cure the disease; rather, the cause remains and lesions may therefore progress elsewhere in the mouth or, subsequently, reoccur as secondary caries near the original sites. A true cure for the disease only takes place when the ionic balance between the loss and uptake of calcium and phosphate ions from the lesion can be made to swing in the overall direction of remineralisation through the implementation of appropriate preventive measures.

Caries is Difficult to Diagnose

Although dentists are the experts at diagnosing caries, it should not be taken for granted that they are infallible. Dental epidemiologists have battled with the issue for years and they have found it necessary to institute comprehensive training programmes for their examiners. In the treatment setting, the size of the problem was demonstrated by a study which reported very wide variation in the diagnoses made by 12 dental school teachers who each examined the same group of 10 patients, and these differences were systematically carried over into the treatment plans[1]. The problem exists in relation to secondary caries as well as to primary caries, as demonstrated in a simulated clinical study where more than a 5-fold variation was found among nine dentists as to which teeth were thought to have caries among a set of 228 extracted teeth[2]. The dentists cannot all have been correct in their diagnoses, therefore most must have been wrong. There was also considerable lack of correspondence between the teeth the dentists considered had caries and those found, after sectioning, to have caries.

Treatment Decisions are Inconsistent

Differences in treatment decisions made by staff and students, or between two members of staff, are well-known to those who work

59

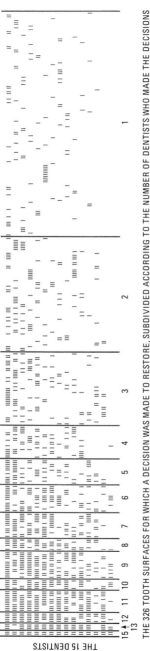

Fig. 9.1 *Diagram showing the decisions to restore that were made by 15 dentists who each examined and planned treatment for the same group of 18 young adults[4]. To simplify presentation of the data, the diagram shows the positive decisions to treat that were made for all the patients together, rather as if there had been one giant individual with 487 teeth. The 15 dentists have been ranked on the vertical axis in descending order according to the total number of surfaces they felt should be treated. The 326 locations on the horizontal axis each represent a specified tooth surface for which a decision was made to restore. Each such decision is shown by a vertical mark, and the 326 tooth surfaces have themselves been ranked according to the number of dentists (subdivided by vertical lines) who made the decisions. It is clear that the variation among the dentists was enormous.*

THE 326 TOOTH SURFACES FOR WHICH A DECISION WAS MADE TO RESTORE, SUBDIVIDED ACCORDING TO THE NUMBER OF DENTISTS WHO MADE THE DECISIONS

THE 15 DENTISTS

in dental schools. Yet, it is all too easy to feel confident in planning routine restorative treatment and for dentists to consider their prescribing patterns to be entirely justified. Indeed, with the dearth of knowledge that exists concerning caries progression (*see* Chapter 3, p. 14), it is not surprising that the criteria indicating the appropriateness of operative intervention in its management are open to considerable debate; certainly, there is no universal agreement within the profession as to what these criteria should be.

This lack of accepted criteria at a time of markedly reducing caries prevalence in the developed countries, partly explains why, in a longitudinal study of treatment based upon the UK 1978 Adult Dental Health Survey, the fillings placed by practitioners bore little relationship to those predicted on the basis of the survey findings[3]. Indeed, it was found that almost twice as many tooth surfaces had been filled in the first year following the survey than had been predicted on the basis of the survey examinations, but that only one-quarter of the tooth surfaces classified in the survey as carious or with failed restorations were among these. It follows that seven-eighths of the surfaces that received fillings had not been identified in the survey as being in need of restoring.

To research the matter further, a study was set up to examine the extent of variation among treatment plans formulated under as near to normal working conditions as possible[4]. When 15 dentists each examined and planned treatment for a group of 18 young adults, the number of positive treatment decisions made by the different dentists ranged from 20 to 153 (Fig. 9.1, p. 59). The inescapable conclusion is that many restorative decisions must be incorrect.

Assessment of Restorations

Reasons for the failure of restorations, given subjectively by clinicians, are extremely variable[5]. Thus, the situation exists, uncomfortable though it might appear to many, that not only is there considerable confusion among dentists as to what constitutes appropriate treatment, but also that dentists are often unable to agree as to what has gone wrong when a restoration fails. So how can the dentist take corrective measures when a restoration is replaced? Often he or she cannot, which explains why freshly replaced occlusal amalgam restorations often carry the stigmata of potential failure to such a degree that it can be predicted that their margins will in time take on similar patterns of breakdown to those that they replaced—but the cavities become larger in the process (Fig. 9.2)[5].

So how do dentists try to assess restorations? Many are accustomed to examining the teeth with a probe. Black[6] wrote in 1936: 'The point (of the probe) should be applied with some pressure and, if it enters the enamel a little, so that a very slight pull is required to remove it, the pit should be marked for a restoration, even though there is no sign of decay'. When examining the margins of restorations, it is suggested that dentists commonly attempt to apply similar criteria to these, marginal defects being assessed as if they were pits and fissures. Thus it appears that a 'catch' by the probe is often considered (erroneously) to provide grounds for replacing a restoration, regardless of the absence of caries (Fig. 9.3, p. 62). Indeed, when dentists examined restored extracted teeth in the simulated clinical study mentioned above[2], it was found that caries was only thought to be present with respect to 46% of the restorations that the dentists felt needed

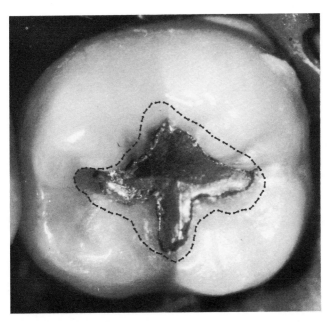

Fig. 9.2 *Lower second molar with an occlusal amalgam restoration that was to be replaced. The dashed line shows the extent of the replacement cavity. There was no caries, but the increase in size is very evident.*

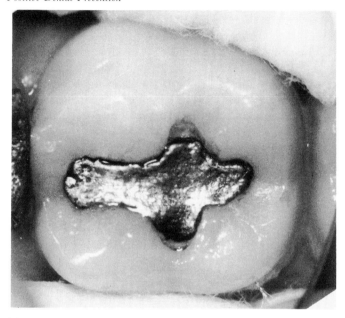

Fig. 9.3 *Example of a lower second molar with an amalgam restoration that has served for some years and which many dentists would consider to be in need of replacement. Certainly a probe would catch at its margins, and there is no doubt that it is morphologically imperfect. But there was no sign of active caries and the patient was not troubled. It was not replaced. (Reproduced by kind permission of A. E. Morgan Publishers of* Restorative Dentistry.*)*

replacing—dentists appear to have (not always justifiably) an urge to replace restorations, and a morphological discrepancy seems to provide this justification. The same conclusion was drawn from a clinical study[7]. However, a morphologically imperfect restoration can be compatible with health and, unless there is caries or the patient is troubled, it is often better to leave the restoration alone—though to monitor it at recall examinations.

DENTAL ATTENDANCE AND RESTORATIONS

In a 5-year study of dental treatment provided for a random sample of dentate adults, it was revealed that the number of tooth surfaces restored over the period went up markedly as the number of courses of treatment rose[8]. It was also noted that the more restorations a person had at the start of the study, the more he or she was likely to receive in the future, for a repeat restorative cycle becomes established. Further, it was found that 50% of the restorative treatment was directed at just 12% of the patients. These people were a high risk group who were at particular risk of having their restorations replaced for, somewhat inevitably, the ratio of replacement restorations to first-time restorations in an individual was found to increase markedly as the overall amount of restorative treatment rose. Indeed, the ratio was over five times greater for patients who received a lot of restorative treatment compared with those who received little restorative treatment, and they were seven times as likely to receive a crown.

This 5-year study also revealed that, among frequently-attending patients, those who changed their dentists at least once, received an average of 13.6 restorations over the period compared with 7.4 for those who stayed with the same dentist[9]. It is clear that the restorative cycle is fuelled by a change of dentist.

IMPLICATIONS

The implications of all these studies are enormous, and it has to be accepted by clinicians that greater caution is required in treatment planning today than is generally thought necessary. By adopting a preventive approach with children and avoiding any unnecessary restorations, there are also enormous additional potential benefits which may not readily be apparent. Thus, an analysis of the dental health status of a group of adults in relation to various psychosocial characteristics has shown that the present restoratively-orientated dental service is offering something that many people do not want, and that it does not offer an acceptable way of meeting their needs[3]. Further, it was concluded from this study that many people who currently avoid dental treatment as much as possible, might come to accept care in a service with a predominantly preventive image. Clearly, it would be shortsighted of any dentist today to manage children in a manner which might exacerbate feelings of dissatisfaction with dentistry; indeed, by offering dental care in a way that makes sense to children and their parents (and prevention makes good sense) it can be expected that there will be an increasing uptake of the dental services in adult life, thereby enhancing the opportunities for preventive dental care in the long term.

REFERENCES

1. Rytomaa I., Jarvinen V., Jarvinen J. (1979). Variation in caries recording and restorative treatment plan among university teachers. *Community Dent. Oral Epidemiol*; **7**: 335–9.
2. Merrett M. C. W., Elderton R. J. (1984). An *in vivo* study of restorative dental treatment decisions and secondary caries. *Brit. Dent. J*; **157**: 128–33.
3. Elderton R. J. (1985). Implications of recent dental health services research on the future of operative dentistry. *J. Public Hlth. Dent*; **45**: 101–5.
4. Elderton R. J., Nuttall N. M. (1983). Variation among dentists in planning treatment. *Brit. Dent. J*; **154**: 201–6.
5. Elderton R. J. (1977). The quality of amalgam restorations. In *Assessment of the Quality of Dental Care*. (Allred H., ed.) pp. 45–81. London: London Hospital Medical College.
6. Black A. D. (1936). *G. V. Black's Work on Operative Dentistry*, Vol. 1, 7th Ed. p. 32. London: Henry Kimpton.
7. Nuttall N. M., Elderton R. J. (1983). The nature of restorative dental treatment decisions. *Brit. Dent. J*; **154**: 363–5.
8. Elderton R. J., Davies J. A. (1984). Restorative dental treatment in the General Dental Service in Scotland. *Brit. Dent. J*; **157**: 196–200.
9. Davies J. A. (1984). The relationship between change of dentist and treatment received in the General Dental Service. *Brit. Dent. J*; **157**: 322–4.

10

Shortcomings of Outdated Restorations and Restorative Procedures

R. J. ELDERTON

Whether in a deciduous or permanent tooth, cavity preparation all too easily involves the removal of large amounts of non-carious enamel and dentine in an endeavour to satisfy outdated interpretations of the principles that were laid down by Black[1] at the beginning of the century.

Unfortunately, Black and generations of authors and teachers to the present day have erroneously led their readers and students to assume that the restorative procedures they describe will normally be successful in the long term. However, the poor durability of average restorations is an established fact, the median life of those placed in a dental service being some 5–10 years[2]. In children, they appear to be very much less durable[3]. If restorations commonly lasted a lifetime, there might be justification for large cavity preparations when small ones would do.

As cavities generally increase in size when restorations are replaced (*see* Fig. 9.2, p. 61), and as teeth become weaker as a result, it is clear that emphasis should be placed upon keeping cavities as small as possible, commensurate with satisfying other requirements. This is the main thrust of the change in thinking on cavity design in recent years.

Discerning textbooks from all parts of the world have advocated an increasingly conservative approach towards cavity preparation. But with few exceptions, all these texts have continued to apply scaled-down interpretations of the old designs, with the result that the cavities advocated are still very mechanistic and the descriptions tend to relate more to hypothetical situations than to teeth with actual carious lesions. A number of distinct problems can be identified.

OUTLINE FORM

The main problem with outdated cavity designs arises from the continued use of Black's term 'outline form'—this has led to the cutting of cavity preparations with preconceived shapes which do not necessarily bear much morphological resemblance to the carious lesions that occasioned them (Figs. 10.1, 10.2).

Black's own interpretation of outline form was that cavity preparations should be cut widely and extended well beyond the extent of the caries, both within the tooth and with respect to the cavity margins. There is a mistaken, yet widely-held, belief that extended preparations with squared-out internal features are essential for allowing a bulk of restorative material and for the

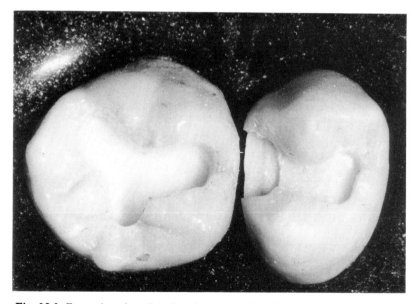

Fig. 10.1 *Examples of outdated cavity preparations for amalgam prepared to rigid outline forms. The caries was minimal, yet the cavities have been cut to about one-third of the intercusp width. They have vertical walls, flat floors and sharply-angled internal features; and they bear little resemblance to the carious lesions that occasioned them.*

prevention of subsequent failure through recurrent caries developing at the margins. However, such restorations have many shortcomings as evidenced by their often poor durability.

One hears to this day, talk of cutting out occlusal fissures to one-third or one-quarter of the intercusp width (Fig. 10.1). But this is neither necessary nor desirable, and it does not stand up to rational thinking. Rather, such considerations serve to epitomise the rigid nature of the way in which outline form is believed and interpreted.

OVERCUTTING

Such a cavity design is very traumatic in that it involves the removal of disproportionately large amounts of sound tooth tissue, partly in order to achieve near-vertical walls, a flat floor and sharp internal line angles (Fig. 10.1)[4]; but why are vertical walls, a flat floor and sharp internal line angles necessary in an occlusal cavity for amalgam or any plastic restorative material? The

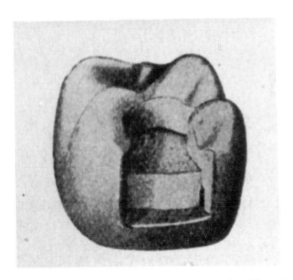

Fig. 10.2 *Drawing of a Black's Class II cavity preparation. Though Black described this as 'the narrow cavity', it has a big angular approximal box which should be seen as a monumental sculpture of a bygone era. Cavity preparations of this type have been responsible for entering many teeth into repeat restoration cycles.* (Reproduced from Black[1].)

answer is that they very definitely are not necessary, and preparations with these characteristics should be condemned. A restoration in a cavity of this type would be obsolescent the day it was placed.

Often the buccal and lingual embrasure walls of an approximo-occlusal cavity preparation are also cut vertically and joined across at the gingival to form a flat floor; but who has seen a carious lesion with a rectangular shape? No-one has, so it must amount to overcutting. Indeed, overcutting is the major problem with the old thinking on Class II cavities—a perceived need for big angular approximal boxes (Fig. 10.2, p. 67)—yet these are both destructive and unnecessary.

CRAZED CERVICAL ENAMEL MARGINS

If the gingival margins of approximal cavities, especially in permanent teeth, are not trimmed appropriately to remove unsupported enamel prisms (which tend to incline gingivally as they pass from the amelodentinal junction towards the surface of the tooth), they are liable to crack and craze as the matrix band is tightened (Fig. 10.3*a* and *b*)[5]. This phenomenon will probably only have been observed by those who use rubber dam (*see* Chapter 12, p. 91), for only then is the enamel able to be dried sufficiently for it to be seen. The complete comedy of errors occurs when a clinician uses a large plugger in an attempt to condense amalgam into an angular approximal 'box' with chipped enamel margins—and in the presence of moisture. Is it any wonder that, at a later date, the restoration will be judged to have secondary caries at the gingival margin and be deemed in need of replacement?

DAMAGE TO THE ADJACENT TOOTH

When preparing Class II cavities, damage to the adjacent tooth appears to be almost universal (Fig. 10.4, p. 70)[6]. While inappropriate cavity preparation technique is responsible, this iatrogenic damage is no doubt exacerbated by the rigours of a perceived need for having to cut sound enamel and dentine when working to old Black-type cavity designs.

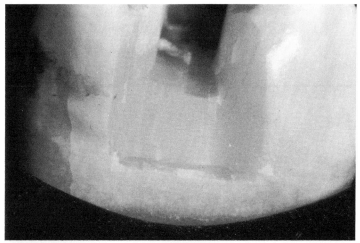

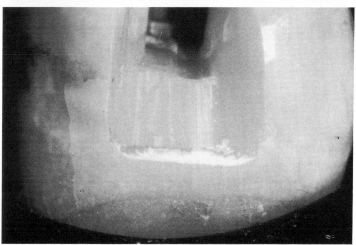

Fig. 10.3a and **b** *Part of the distal surface of an upper premolar in which a 'Black' type cavity has been prepared, but with an inadequately finished cervical margin. a = Before application of a matrix band. b = After application and removal of a matrix band. Note the crazing at the cervical margin that has produced a mass of white enamel chips.* (Reproduced by kind permission of the Editor of the *British Dental Journal*.)

If severe, this damage must jeopardise interproximal cleaning and hence long-term periodontal health; and in a proportion of instances it is likely to lead to caries in the damaged tooth or lead to a perceived need to place a restoration at the damaged site.

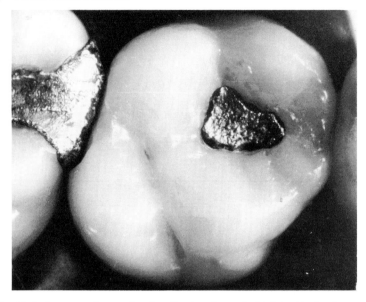

Fig. 10.4 *An upper first molar, the distal surface of which had been damaged extensively by the dentist who, previously, had prepared the MO cavity in the adjacent second molar. At the time this photograph was taken, there was caries in the damaged surface, which extended well into the dentine.*

WEAK AMALGAM MARGINS

With near-vertical cavity walls in an occlusal cavity, the edge of the amalgam that will be adapted to them is bound to be thin and weak (Fig. 10.5), and therefore liable to breakdown (Fig. 10.6, p. 72). Indeed, it has been shown that the edge angle of an occlusal amalgam restoration should be of at least 70° on the occlusal surface if the margins are to stand a good chance of not breaking down in function at an early stage[7]. By preparing the cavity walls in the general long axis of the crown, the potential for an amalgam margin angle anywhere near 70° is compromised severely. This type of cavity design cannot, therefore, be satisfactory and it should be discontinued.

POORLY-FITTING AMALGAM MARGINS

It has also been found with this type of design that the precise

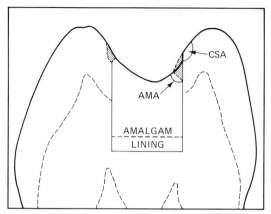

Fig. 10.5 *Diagrammatic bucco-lingual section through a posterior tooth with an outdated cavity preparation and a freshly-placed amalgam restoration illustrating common faults. The cavo-surface angles (CSA) are too high and the amalgam margin angles (AMA) are too low, leaving the amalgam edges thin and weak. On the right side, the amalgam has erroneously been finished short of the cavity margin (marked S in Fig. 10.7, p. 72). Gradual fracturing of this amalgam edge in function would be very likely, leaving a ditched margin as indicated by the stippled area. On the left, excess amalgam has erroneously been left as flash in a concave region of the occlusal surface (such as a secondary fissure—marked E in Fig. 10.7). This excess would be likely to break off in function, leaving a ditched margin and an apparent marginal defect of the proportions shown by the stippling. This diagram is based upon tracings produced from an* in vivo *study[7].*

position of the cavity margin becomes difficult to see clinically and to work to, with the result that the restoration is commonly over- or under-carved at the time it is placed, and is therefore often a misfit with the cavity preparation (Fig. 10.7, p. 72)[8]. These misfits have the effect of increasing the size of the defects that form as marginal breakdown takes place (see the stippled areas in Fig. 10.5).

Surprisingly, however, clinicians are remarkably unaware of these problems; indeed, it has been noted that clinicians are usually very satisfied with restorations they have just placed, even when they contain these very characteristics of in-built obsolescence[8]. This feeling of a 'job well done' partly explains why these old cavity designs continue to be perpetuated—many dentists do not realise that they are wrong.

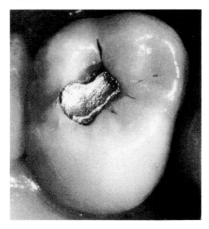

Fig. 10.6 *Occlusal amalgam restoration in an upper molar where marginal breakdown has taken place through the mechanism described for the right side in Fig. 10.5 (p. 71). As there was no sign of caries and no symptoms, the restoration was not replaced.*

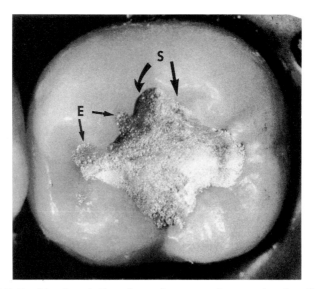

Fig. 10.7 *Freshly-placed, though mediocre, amalgam restoration that was placed in the cavity illustrated in Fig. 9.2 (p. 61). The amalgam was, in places, in excess (E) and in places short (S) of the cavity margin. There is little doubt that the amalgam margin angle was too low in most regions, so the mechanisms of marginal failure illustrated in Fig. 10.5 (p. 71) can be expected to operate.*

REFERENCES

1. Black G. V. (1908). *A Work on Operative Dentistry*. Vol. 2. pp. 110–6. Chicago: The Medico-Dental Publishing Co.
2. Elderton R. J. (1983). Longitudinal study of dental treatment in the General Dental Service in Scotland. *Brit. Dent. J*; **155**: 91–6.
3. Holland I. S., Walls A. W. G., Wallwork M. A., Murray J. J. (1986). The longevity of amalgam restorations in deciduous molars. *Brit. Dent. J*; **161**: 225–8.
4. Elderton R. J. (1986). Restorative dentistry: 1. Current thinking on cavity design. *Dent. Update*; **13**: 113–22, 240.
5. Elderton R. J. (1984). New approaches to cavity design with special reference to the Class II lesion. *Brit. Dent. J*; **157**: 421–7.
6. Cardwell J. E., Roberts B. J. (1972). Damage to adjacent teeth during cavity preparation. *J. Dent. Res*; **51**: 1269–70.
7. Elderton R. J. (1984). Cavo-surface angles, amalgam margin angles and occlusal cavity preparations. *Brit. Dent. J*; **156**: 319–24.
8. Elderton R. J. (1975). An *in vivo* morphological study of cavity and amalgam margins on the occlusal surfaces of human teeth. PhD thesis. London: University of London.

11

Preventive Management of Dental Caries

R. J. ELDERTON

Like all health professionals, dentists are inherently cautious about overlooking the possibility of disease, and the unwritten maxim for some still appears to be: 'If in doubt, fill or refill', yet 'if in doubt, prevent, wait and reassess' would be more in keeping with the requirements of modern dentistry.

When assessing carious lesions, the crucial issue from the management point of view is not to answer the somewhat academic question: 'Is there caries?' but to answer the more practical questions: 'Is there *active* caries?' and if so, 'Can it be arrested?'

When examining for carious lesions and assessing their extent and activity, good visualisation is important. While a probe may be useful for removing superficial debris and plaque from the site, no attempt should ever be made to penetrate a possible lesion. Probing may penetrate the highly mineralised zone of an early carious lesion and reach the decalcified sub-surface layer, thereby enhancing the breakdown of the partly decalcified tissues[1], presumably rendering them less capable of remineralisation. Certainly, whether or not a lesion is sticky on probing is irrelevant to the question of whether or not it is active. If there is no cavitation probing achieves nothing, whereas if there is cavitation, it is rare that the lesion cannot also be seen. Very early approximal cavitation, or approximal cavitation where there are very broad contacts, may be exceptions.

Professional participation in encouraging the arresting process with respect to a smooth surface lesion usually requires different management from that at a pit or fissure site[2].

SMOOTH SURFACE LESIONS

While fastidious application of the full gamut of preventive measures would cause any and every lesion to arrest (*see* Plates 4 and 5), a compromise situation normally prevails, for only a limited uptake of prevention usually occurs. However, even small changes in dietary habits, a moderate increase in the use of fluoride materials, or a little additional attention to plaque removal, might be sufficient to tip the balance towards remineralisation and arrest. It is realistic to use mirrors to show the lesion to the patient and parent and to encourage particular attention to oral hygiene with respect to the specific site where the lesion is located. Dietary advice should be given, and the patient encouraged to ensure that fluoride toothpaste is regularly applied directly to the lesion. For approximal lesions, interdental flossing every day or two would seem sensible. How can a Class II lesion be expected to arrest when plaque lies constantly against it?

The Decision to Restore (*see* Chapter 12)

Which smooth surface lesions is it realistic to attempt to arrest and which should be restored? There is no clear-cut answer, but, with the present state of knowledge, there are certain conditions concerning Class II, III and V lesions which usually indicate that a restoration is required in a permanent tooth. These include:

- the tooth is sensitive to hot, cold, sweetness, etc;
- the lesion can be judged to have spread at least half way through the dentine (Figs. 11.1, 11.2, pp. 76, 77) (sometimes it is appropriate to restore when a lesion is considerably less advanced than this, but knowledge is lacking in this area);
- the pulp is thought to be in jeopardy of becoming involved before the next dental examination;
- previous attempts to arrest the lesion have failed and there is evidence that the lesion is progressing (such evidence usually requires an observation period of months or years);
- function is impaired;
- drifting is likely to occur through loss of a contact point;
- aesthetic reasons.

Similar criteria apply to deciduous teeth assuming, of course, that exfoliation is not just around the corner.

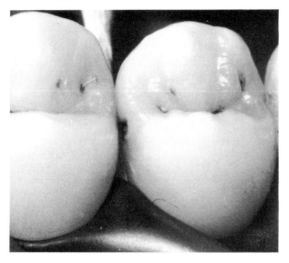

Fig. 11.1 *An upper premolar for which a bitewing radiograph indicated that the mesial carious lesion had penetrated half way through the dentine. Open cavitation is clearly evident, and a restoration was deemed appropriate for this patient.* (Reproduced by kind permission of A. E. Morgan, Publishers of *Restorative Dentistry*.)

The Decision to Arrest

When none of the above conditions apply, the most professional approach to Class II, III and V lesions would often seem to be as follows (Fig. 11.2):

- record the site of the lesion;
- demonstrate its presence to the patient and/or parent, using mirrors, etc;
- institute a general preventive programme together with personalised preventive measures that are relevant to the particular lesion;
- say to the patient and/or parent: 'It is largely up to you, for it is you who will apply the preventive measures'.
- arrange to reassess the lesion with the patient at recall intervals (*see* Chapter 4, p. 26) and reinforce the preventive measures or, if it seems appropriate at that time, restore as necessary.

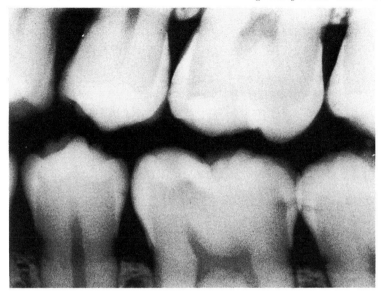

Fig. 11.2 *Bitewing radiograph showing caries in the distal and occlusal sur-*
faces of the lower first molar which appears to have spread at least half way
through the dentine at both sites. Restoration at this time, together with the
implementation of preventive measures, would be the correct treatment. By
comparison, it would not necessarily be appropriate to restore the mesial
lesion in the lower second molar at this time, for this is much smaller. It
should be reassessed at recall intervals, for, in view of preventive measures,
it may not progress. Arresting of the early mesial lesions in the upper first
molar and in the distal of the lower second premolar should certainly be
prime objectives in the dental care of this patient.

PIT AND FISSURE LESIONS

Because it is often difficult to assess accurately the status of small
pit and fissure lesions, it is inevitable that monitoring them over
time is fraught with danger. It would therefore seem inappropriate to adopt any type of watch-and-wait approach, even if maximum use is also made of home preventive measures and topical
fluoride applications.

If there is clear evidence of cavitation involving the dentine, or if
caries in the dentine can be observed on a bitewing radiograph
(Fig. 3.3, p. 18), an invasive restorative procedure would seem
warranted. The choice would normally lie between an amalgam

or a composite resin restoration (or glass-ionomer cement or silver cermet in a deciduous tooth) in a modern minimal cavity preparation (*see* Chapter 12, p. 82) using a sealant restoration technique if appropriate.

If the lesion is small or there is doubt as to its presence or activity (the questionable lesion) (Fig. 11.3*a* and *b*), a non-invasive method of management is the only one that ensures no over-treatment. However, it is inappropriate to leave such pits and fissures alone; the application of fissure sealant to them provides the only realistic solution, and an excellent one at that.

Fissure Sealants

Fissure sealants have been used widely and successfully to prevent dental caries for some 20 years[3], and the American Dental Association[4] in 1983 considered them safe and effective as a caries preventive procedure. Their efficacy has recently been endorsed by the Joint British Dental Association/Department of Health and Social Security Working Party on Fissure Sealants[5].

Sealants as a primary preventive measure. Sealing all pits and fissures as the teeth erupt, for the whole population of children as a primary preventive measure for sound untreated teeth, cannot be justified on economic and logistical grounds; indeed, such a regime could be considered to amount to over-treatment. Such over use could even result in the initiation of caries and/or an invasive restorative procedure (*see* Plate 6). The use of fissure sealant as a primary preventive measure is, however, recommended under certain conditions (and as part of an overall preventive package) including:

- for teeth considered to be at special risk of becoming carious, e.g.:
  —in caries-prone individuals;
  —in teeth contralateral to those that have already become carious;
  —in teeth that have habitually plaque-covered fissured surfaces (*see* Plates 7, 8);
- for patients whose dental and/or general health is compromised by circumstances which render them especially at risk from dental disease or treatment, or for whom more invasive forms of dental treatment may present particular

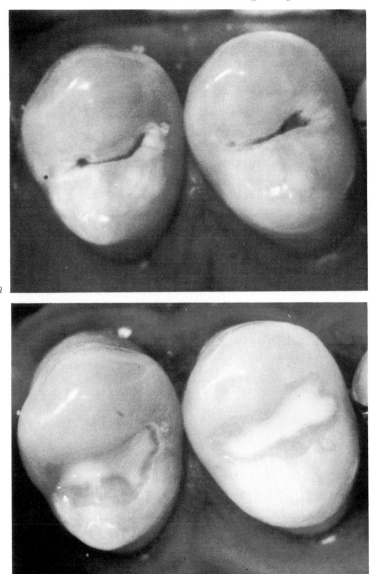

Fig. 11.3a and **b** *Upper premolars that were judged as caries-free 2 years previously, but which were thought at the time of the photographs, probably to have small active fissure lesions (as opposed to staining only). a = Before fissure sealing. b = After application of the sealant.* (Reproduced by kind permission of the Editor of the *British Dental Journal.*)

problems (e.g. mentally or physically handicapped individuals, haemophiliacs).

Sealants as a therapeutic treatment for caries. There is considerable research evidence to support the efficacy of applying fissure sealant therapeutically to early pit and fissure lesions to arrest the caries[3]. Indeed, many millions of early carious lesions in pits and fissures must have been sealed over in good faith by dentists who, at the time, considered the surfaces to be sound; and the sealant appears to have worked. Fissure sealants have also been tested as a therapeutic treatment of more advanced carious lesions (shown radiographically to extend up to half way through the dentine)[3]. The author has not found a single report of caries having been shown to have progressed at a pit or fissure site where fissure sealant had remained intact over a carious lesion in a clinical study. The sealant has the effect of dramatically reducing the viable bacterial flora to a level which is too low to enable the caries to progress. The carious material assumes characteristics which are compatible with those of arrested caries, and it seems ultimately that the lesions may become sterile. Some remineralisation of the carious dentine may occur. The use of fissure sealant as a preventive/therapeutic treatment is, therefore, appropriate under the following circumstances:

- for teeth judged to have *active* early pit or fissure caries (*see* Plates 2, 3);
- for teeth judged to have early pit or fissure caries, but where the activity of the disease is in doubt (Fig. 11.3, p. 79).
- for 'don't know' situations where the dentist is in doubt and unable to decide as to whether a small carious lesion is present or not. With respect to the pits and fissures, this supports the maxim 'if in doubt, seal'.

It will be appreciated that these criteria apply equally to the deciduous and permanent dentitions, and to all pitted or fissured tooth surfaces (i.e. including palatal surfaces of upper incisors, wisdom teeth, etc). However, the technique is inappropriate where a pit or fissure is in a relatively unprotected site, such as near a marginal ridge (*see* Plate 9). Here, an invasive restorative procedure would be more appropriate. With deciduous teeth, glass-ionomer cement appears to have a special place as a fissure sealant on account of the chemical nature of the bonding mechanism.

It will be realised that the therapeutic use of fissure sealant may be the only realistic treatment option for a pit or fissure lesion in an uncooperative patient.

REFERENCES

1. Bergman G., Linden L-A. (1969). The action of the explorer on incipient caries. *Svensk. Tandl. Tids*; **62**: 629–34.
2. Elderton R. J. (1985). Assessment and clinical management of early caries in young adults: invasive versus non-invasive methods. *Brit. Dent. J*; **185**: 440–4.
3. Elderton R. J. (1985). Management of early dental caries in fissures with fissure sealant. *Brit. Dent. J*; **158**: 254–8.
4. American Dental Association Council on Dental Materials, Instruments and Equipment. (1983). Pit and fissure sealants. *J. Amer. Dent. Ass*; **107**: 465.
5. Dowell T. B., Elderton R. J., Cole P., *et al.* (1986). Fissure sealants. Report of the Joint BDA/DHSS Working Party. *Brit. Dent. J*; **161**: 343–4.

12

Preventively-orientated Restorations and Restorative Procedures

R. J. ELDERTON

In permanent teeth, restorations (realistically, a series of restorations) are normally intended to last a lifetime. To fulfil a preventive function in terms of dental health in adult life, restorative procedures should, therefore, be undertaken with extreme care and finesse, with only the most suitable materials being used. As cavity preparation is an irreversible procedure, tissue cut away unnecessarily is likely to compromise a successful and trouble-free result in the long term.

When considering deciduous teeth, it should be appreciated that many restorations are required for 5–10 years, which happens to be similar to the median survival time of routine amalgam restorations in permanent teeth in adults. As restorations have been shown to be even *less* durable in deciduous teeth, it is clear that at least equal care is required in their execution. With deciduous teeth, there do, however, appear to be good reasons for considering glass-ionomer cement or silver cermet as alternatives to amalgam for restorations involving the occlusal surfaces (*see* Chapter 13, p. 95). In their present state of development, they cannot, however, be recommended as routine restorative materials for the occlusal surfaces of permanent teeth.

THE PREVENTIVE APPROACH TO CAVITY DESIGN

Dentistry today requires a modern, preventive, approach to cavity design. With this, the over-riding aim is the removal of the carious tissue and unsupported enamel, rather than the cutting of an outline form *per se*. The finished cavity then very much resembles the shape of the carious lesion it replaces but, where necessary, includes refinements, such as the removal of radiating fissures to satisfy other requirements. These requirements should be based upon rational logic aimed at leaving the tooth maximally strong.

Small cavity preparations can be expected to be associated with less trauma to the pulp; and small restorations are easier to retain and lesser occlusal forces are applied to them. They may be more aesthetic than larger ones. They are also more likely to be shaped to reproduce the anatomy of the missing tissue. This means that they are less likely to cause any alteration of inter-arch or intra-arch relationships, or to disturb normal gingival health. Most importantly, should a small restoration fail, there will be more tooth tissue left in which to make a replacement restoration, than would have been the case if the previous one had already been large.

CLASS I CAVITY FOR AMALGAM

The optimum occlusal cavity preparation for amalgam, using present-day technology, has its widest part determined by the spread of the caries at the amelodentinal junction (Fig. 12.1*a* and *b*, p. 84). Where the cusps are steeply inclined, the cavo-surface angles should be cut to a compromise of about 105° to enable the amalgam edges to be thick and strong, with amalgam margin angles of at least the critical 70° which is necessary to given them a good chance of withstanding function[1].

Cavo-surface angles of this order are consistent with leaving the enamel margins strong and they are sufficiently well-defined to enhance good adaptation of the amalgam. This part of the cavity is readily cut with a fine tapered fissure bar.

The floor of the cavity in the wide part of the cavity takes the form of the natural curve that is left behind after excavating the carious dentine. This part of the cavity will, of course, be covered with lining material, which further nullifies any argument for cutting away even more to make it flat.

Where the cavity has to be extended to remove a V-shaped fissure (for amalgam cannot be well adapted to such a fissure

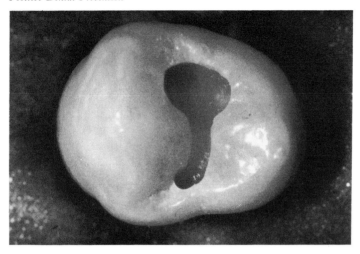

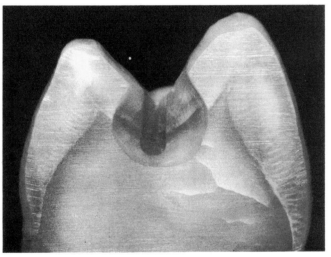

Fig. 12.1a and **b** *Occlusal view of an upper premolar with a correct cavity preparation for amalgam. The cavity has been prepared as if there had been a considerable spread of caries at one end, but only minimal caries in the fissure at the other. a = Occlusal view. b = Bucco-lingual section through the wide region of the cavity. The preparation is widest at the amelodentinal junction, and the enamel walls have been cut to produce cavo-surface angles of about 105°–110°. For a tooth such as this with steeply-sloping cusps, these angles represent a realistic compromise between what is ideal and what is possible. The narrow part of the cavity can be seen in the background in profile.* (Reproduced by kind permission of the Editor of the British Dental Journal.)

when it radiates from a cavity), a single sweep of a Jet 330 bur produces a preparation that is just undercut and no more than 0.8 mm wide. This is about one-eighth of the intercusp width of a premolar. As there is never any occlusal interference in these regions, the all-important high amalgam margin angles are produced (with room to spare) by carving the amalgam flat in these narrow parts (Fig. 12.2).

These principles apply to all Class I cavities for amalgam, irrespective of the teeth or surfaces involved, providing the caries does not undermine a cusp tip, in which case the cusp tip would have to be included in the restoration and amalgam would sometimes then be an inappropriate restorative material. With a permanent tooth, cast gold or composite resin might be more satisfactory, whereas with a deciduous tooth, a preformed stainless steel crown would often be the restoration of choice (*see* Chapter 13, p. 95).

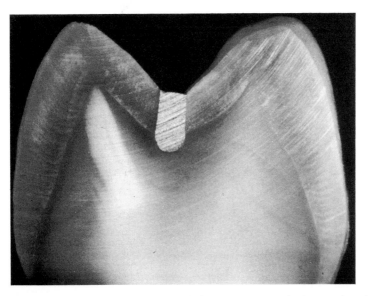

Fig. 12.2 *Bucco-lingual section through the narrow part of a restored cavity similar to that shown in Fig. 12.1. The cavo-surface angles are high, but the amalgam margins are strong because they have been carved flat. (Reproduced by kind permission of the Editor of the* British Dental Journal.)

CLASS I CAVITY FOR COMPOSITE RESIN OR GLASS-IONOMER CEMENT

Acid etch-retained composite resin has a particular advantage over amalgam as a restorative material for occlusal cavities where a combined sealant restoration technique (preventive resin restoration) can be used. Such a situation would be where caries-free or minimally carious V-shaped fissures radiate away from the site of a carious lesion that itself warrants excision and restoration (Fig. 12.3)[2]. This is a very conservative method of treating pit or fissure caries that is other than minimal (in which case fissure sealant would be used—*see* Chapter 11, p. 78) or which has spread to an unknown extent into the dentine (*see* Plate 9).

Where a lesion is patently obvious, cavity preparation for the

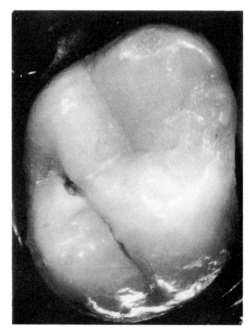

Fig. 12.3 *Upper second molar with a substantial active carious lesion centred on the distal occlusal pit. The occluso-lingual fissure was judged to have early active caries. A sealant restoration, whereby the main carious lesion is excised and restored with acid etch-retained composite resin and the occluso-lingual fissure sealed, would be ideal.* (Reproduced by kind permission of A. E. Morgan, Publishers of *Restorative Dentistry*.)

new plastic materials is the same as for when amalgam is to be used except, of course, that some fissures are not excised. Where the size of the lesion is unknown, an exploratory excavation of the carious pit or fissure is made initially with a small round bur and the extent of the lesion at the amelodentinal junction is assessed. Where caries is present, the cavity is then enlarged as necessary, as described above for amalgam (Fig. 12.4). If a mis-diagnosis should prove to have been made, the procedure should be aborted and the sealant restoration placed at that stage.

The same principles apply when using glass-ionomer cement or silver cermet in deciduous teeth, though being a rather viscous material, many clinicians advise the use of the smallest round bur to widen any fissures that are to be sealed with these materials. Some clinicians have reported excellent success with glass-ionomer cement used in this way as a primary preventive measure for fissured surfaces of permanent teeth, the material being pressed into the widened fissures with finger pressure over 'cling' film.

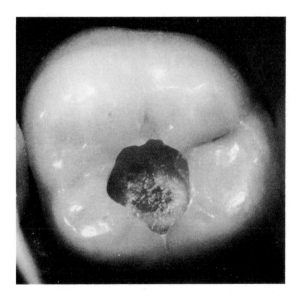

Fig. 12.4 *The tooth shown in Plate 9 after opening up the carious lesion and making the amelodentinal junction caries-free. The tooth was restored with amalgam, but if there had been V-shaped fissures extending from the cavity, an acid etch-retained sealant restoration would have been appropriate.*

CLASS II CAVITY FOR AMALGAM

The above principles apply precisely to Class II cavity preparations. The shape of the approximal part of the completed cavity
takes on a rounded form commensurate with the shape of the
carious lesion (Fig. 12.5). Apart from the region of the marginal
ridge through which access is made to the lesion, this shape is
determined entirely by the spread of the caries at the amelodentinal junction, and it is mapped out with a slowly rotating round bur
which is moved back and forth along this junction until it is free of
caries[3].

It is generally optimum for the buccal and lingual cavity margins to lie just out of contact with the adjacent tooth. A hair's
breadth of clearance is all that is required, though the spread of
the caries will often dictate a wider preparation.

It is irrational to extend the cervical part of the cavity into the

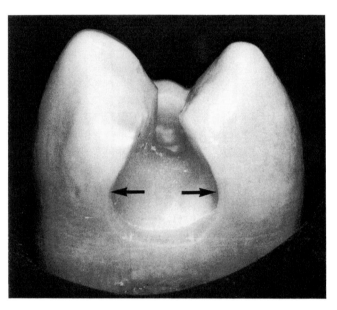

Fig. 12.5 *Modern optimum Class II cavity for amalgam in an upper premolar
where there had been a large approximal carious lesion but minimal
occlusal caries. As far as possible, the cavity has been prepared according
to the shape and extent of the carious lesion. Approximal retention grooves
(arrowed) serve to hold the restoration in place, thereby preventing any
tendency for fracturing of the amalgam in the region of the marginal ridge.*

gingival crevice, for such areas are no longer believed to be immune from secondary caries, and gingival irritation is likely to be caused by so doing. Subgingival margins are less easy to manage clinically, and they are less amenable to subsequent re-evaluation. With rounded, minimally extended cavities, the chances of adapting a well-fitting matrix band are much greater than when the embrasure walls of the cavity have been cut widely and squarely.

To prevent the amalgam from being displaced through occlusal forces, the dentine part of the gingival floor of the cavity should incline inwards slightly in a mesio-distal plane, so that the amalgam tends to get pushed into the cavity under occlusal loading. Grooves should also be placed in the dentine of the buccal and lingual embrasure walls to provide independent retention for the approximal surface of the restoration, thereby precluding any possibility of a tendency for the occlusal and approximal parts of the restoration to separate (i.e. preventing fracture in the region of

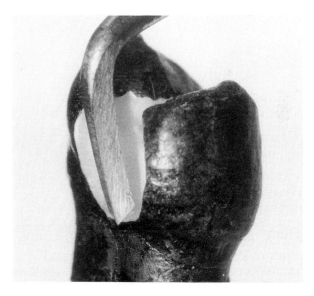

Fig. 12.6 *A gingival margin trimmer being used to finish the enamel margin of a Class II cavity so that unsupported enamel prisms are not left in situ. If they are, crazing of the margin could occur subsequently as shown in Fig. 10.3 p. 69). The surface of this tooth has been stained darkly to enhance contrast.* (Reproduced by kind permission of the Editor of the *British Dental Journal.*)

the marginal ridge) (Fig. 12.5, p. 88). This being so, it is not
necessary to have a wide or deep occlusal keyway; indeed, the only
purpose of the occlusal extension to the cavity should be to remove
the occlusal fissure where necessary.

In order to avoid damaging the adjacent tooth, the removal of
carious and unsupported enamel at the periphery of the approximal part of the cavity, once the amelodentinal junction is caries
free, requires careful attention to detail. Unless there is no tooth
adjacent, this stage is best accomplished with a sharp gingival
margin trimmer (Fig. 12.6, p. 89)[3].

This instrument is first used as a hatchet to cut the embrasure
wall of the cavity in a gingival direction from the marginal ridge.
Then, reversing the action, it is swept along the gingival part of
the cavity margin and up the embrasure wall, chipping off loose
enamel as it goes, thereby, at the same time, eliminating the
possibility of a crazed gingival margin subsequently when the
matrix band is tightened against the tooth (*see* Fig. 10.3, p. 69).
This method will not damage the adjacent tooth, unlike the
situation when a bur is used to prepare and finish these margins.

CLASS II CAVITY FOR COMPOSITE RESIN OR GLASS-IONOMER CEMENT

With acid etch-retained composite resin or glass-ionomer cement
(the latter in deciduous teeth only) the approximal part of the
cavity should be prepared precisely as for amalgam. The occlusal
part has been described above, and it will be appreciated that the
sealant restoration technique is a variant that should be used
whenever appropriate.

The internal or tunnel preparation for glass-ionomer cement or
silver cermet is being used increasingly for Class II carious
lesions[4]. With this method, access to the lesion is made through
the occlusal surface of the tooth leaving the marginal ridge intact,
and the restorative material is injected into the cavity through this
approach. In combination with a composite resin overlay[5] on the
occlusal surface of the glass-ionomer material (serving also as a
fissure sealant, as necessary), this may prove to be an efficacious
way of maintaining as much sound tooth tissue as possible. Long-
term clinical results of using this method are awaited with
interest.

GENERAL

Use of the word 'conservative' should not necessarily be interpreted as being synonymous with 'small'—clearly, a small cavity preparation is not possible when the carious lesion is large, though it can and should be as small as possible commensurate with complete removal of all the caries at the amelodentinal junction. Indeed, it should be stressed that in striving for conservative cavity preparations, caries should never be left at the amelodentinal junction. It is, however, normally a better option to leave very deep caries lying close to the pulp in teeth considered not to have irreversible pulpitis, than to expose the pulp in an endeavour to excavate every last trace of the caries in this part of the cavity. A calcium hydroxide lining material should be placed over any such deep caries that is left *in situ*.

It is advantageous to use rubber dam for most cavity preparations and restorations. With the rubber dam in place, there is complete control over the cheeks, lips, tongue and gingiva, thereby enhancing visibility and access to the teeth, especially when working at the back of the mouth or near the gingival tissue. This enables more accurate scrutiny of the extent of carious lesions and of the exact configuration of fissure patterns, etc. Accurate tooth preparation is easier to achieve and cavity detail is much more evident. When operating upon carious lesions near the gingiva, the rubber dam is really the only way of achieving even adequate isolation, let alone the perfect field that can usually be achieved.

The physical properties of all dental materials are enhanced if they are used in their pure and uncontaminated forms, and this itself is sufficient reason to warrant applying a rubber dam for all restorations. Indeed, with the newer restorative materials, including glass-ionomer cements and acid-etch retained composite resins, the cleanliness of the field, only made possible by the rubber dam, may be seen as essential. Then, when matrix bands are removed after placing an approximal restoration, an onslaught of blood and saliva to obscure the restoration margins cannot occur. Indeed, there is a greatly enhanced possibility of actually being able to see the embrasure and gingival margins, and consequently to carve them to excellent contour. Proper adaptation of the restorative material in these critical regions can also be checked. In a nutshell, restorative dentistry is simplified with a rubber dam in place.

The rubber dam also has many other advantages. It enhances the control of cross-infection, and it allows the patient to be much more relaxed during dental procedures. The patient is, however, still quite capable of communicating adequately with the dentist, and the rubber dam works well with children. Correct technique of application[6] is the key to its successful use.

REFERENCES

1. Elderton R. J. (1984). Cavo-surface angles, amalgam margin angles and occlusal cavity preparations. *Brit. Dent. J*; **156**: 319–24.
2. Simonsen R. J. (1982). Potential uses of pit-and-fissure sealants in innovative ways: a review. *J. Publ. Hlth. Dent*; **42**: 305–11.
3. Elderton R. J. (1984). New approaches to cavity design with special reference to the Class II lesion. *Brit. Dent. J*; **157**: 421–7.
4. McLean J. W., Gasser O. (1985). Glass-cermet cements. *Quint. Int*; **16**: 333–43.
5. McLean J. W., Prosser H. J., Wilson A. D. (1985). The use of glass-ionomer cements in bonding composite resins to dentine. *Brit. Dent. J*; **158**: 410–14.
6. Elderton R. J. (1971). A modern approach to the use of rubber dam. *Dent. Pract. Dent. Rec*; **21**: 187–93, 226–32, 267–73.

13

Special Considerations in the Restoration of Deciduous Teeth

J. J. MURRAY

RATIONALE FOR RESTORING DECIDUOUS TEETH

The idea that, because deciduous teeth are 'temporary' there is no need to restore them, should have been discarded decades ago. However, because of the limited life span of deciduous teeth it is sometimes appropriate to use different restorative materials than for permanent teeth. The main reasons for restoring deciduous teeth are:

- to prevent pain;
- to reduce the need for extractions;
- to prevent complications of crowding in the permanent dentition.

The 1983 Children's Dental Health Survey[1] revealed that 27% of 8-year-olds had had at least one general anaesthetic for the removal of (mostly deciduous) teeth. While this is a marked improvement from the figure of 49% for the same group in 1973, it is still a horrendous figure. Indeed, the removal of carious deciduous teeth is the major reason for the administration of a general anaesthetic to a child in Great Britain. Of the 400 000 general anaesthetics given in the General Dental Service in England and Wales in 1984, three-quarters were administered to children under 16 years of age.

The early loss of a deciduous molar will not, *per se*, cause crowding, but in a child with a tendency to crowding, the loss of one or more deciduous molars will allow the first permanent molar in the affected quadrant(s) to move mesially, often tilting and rotating in the process, thereby concentrating the site of the crowding to the premolar region and perhaps causing a midline deviation (*see* Chapter 14, p. 104). Both complicate orthodontic treatment.

All the principles of caries management and cavity preparation with respect to the permanent teeth apply equally to the deciduous dentition. The preventively-minded dentist will, however, appreciate certain differences in restorative treatment.

DECIDUOUS INCISORS AND CANINES

Children with caries in anterior deciduous teeth must be considered caries-prone, and glass-ionomer cement, with its fluoride-leaching characteristic, is therefore the restorative material of choice. Clearly, labial lesions in these teeth should not be restored without first identifying (and endeavouring to eliminate) the bad habits that predisposed to their occurrence. In some cases, the removal of the aetiological factor prevents further disintegration of the affected teeth, and the correct use of fluoride toothpaste is all that is required to maintain these teeth until exfoliation (*see* Plate 5).

DECIDUOUS MOLARS

While amalgam has traditionally been the dental material used to restore Class II cavities in the molars, little information is available concerning the longevity of amalgam restorations in these teeth, though in a recent study of 1139 such restorations, the median survival time was estimated to be 31 months[2]. The age of the child at the time of placement had an important effect on the durability of the restoration: the median survival time was only 11 months in the youngest age group (3 years of age) increasing to 44 months for children aged 7–8 years.

Obviously patient cooperation, the ability of the operator, the type of cavity preparation and the use of local analgesia, all play a part in the longevity of the restoration. However, deciduous teeth are subject to a great deal of attrition and abrasion, and sometimes it appears that occlusal factors are the cause of the failure and that the tooth structure itself fails around the amalgam restoration. For this reason, glass-ionomer cements or silver cermets, which bond chemically to the tooth, may well have a part to play in the future[3]. In a prospective study comparing the performance of these cements with amalgam in pairs of deciduous molar teeth, no difference in the overall failure rate of the two materials was found over 2 years, nor was there any differences in the rate of loss of marginal integrity[4]. The glass-ionomer restorations did, however, show a greater loss of anatomical form during the early stages of the follow up period.

It is not possible to say whether current glass-ionomer cements or silver cermets are sufficiently satisfactory to supersede amalgam as a restorative material for deciduous molars, as their flexural strength is not, theoretically, satisfactory for stress-bearing areas. However, many clinicians are very enthusiastic about their use for this purpose, and they certainly offer attractive possibilities for the future.

Where a deciduous molar has a moderately-sized carious lesion or when endodontic treatment has been carried out, a correctly placed preformed stainless steel or nickel-chrome crown[5] provides an excellent restoration; these should be in routine use by all dentists undertaking restorative treatment for children.

REFERENCES

1. Todd J. E., Dodd T. (1985). *Children's Dental Health in the United Kingdom 1983*. London: HMSO.
2. Holland I. S., Walls A. W. G., Wallwork M. A., Murray J. J. (1986). The longevity of amalgam restorations in deciduous molars. *Brit. Dent. J*; **161**: 255–8.
3. Croll T. P., Phillips R. W. (1986). Glass ionomer-silver cermet restorations for primary teeth. *Quint. Int*; **17**: 607–15.
4. Walls A. W. G. (1986). A clinical and laboratory investigation of adhesive restorative materials. PhD Thesis. Newcastle: University of Newcastle upon Tyne.
5. Brook A. H., King N. M. (1982). The role of stainless steel crowns. Part I—properties and technique. *Dental Update*; **Jan/Feb**: 25–30.

14

Extractions as a Preventive Measure

I. D. BROWN

One or more timely extractions should sometimes be seen as a powerful preventive measure for the dentition as a whole and for long-term dental health. It is important that all dentists are aware of the situations when such planned extractions are beneficial.

SERIAL EXTRACTION

Parents frequently ask whether anything can be done to resolve the crowding of their child's recently erupted permanent incisors. The relief of crowding usually has to await the eruption of the first premolars. However, in very carefully selected cases, the technique of serial extraction can be commenced at about 8 years of age when the mandibular lateral incisors are erupting. Serial extraction can produce good results where:

- there is a Class I occlusion with mild crowding in both arches;
- none of the permanent incisors are rotated;
- the first premolars are developmentally ahead of the canines;
- the first permanent molars have a good prognosis;
- all the permanent teeth, with the possible exception of third molars, are present.

The first step is to extract the four deciduous canines when the mandibular lateral incisors are erupting so that the incisor crowding can resolve at the expense of space for the permanent canines. The four deciduous first molars are then extracted 1 year later to ensure that the first premolars erupt in advance of the canines. Lastly, the four first premolars are extracted in order to provide space for the erupting canines.

This sequence sounds very convincing in theory, but in practice it is often found that the desired spontaneous tooth movements do not occur; for example, the canines may erupt before the first premolars. It is worth noting that warning comments concerning serial extractions have been included in two recent orthodontic textbooks[1,2]. For any particular patient, this form of treatment should be chosen with care, and unless the dentist is experienced, referral of the patient for confirmatory advice is mandatory. The alternative to serial extraction is to delay treatment for the relief of crowding until the first premolars and canines have erupted.

MANAGEMENT OF PATIENTS WITH ONE OR MORE FIRST PERMANENT MOLARS OF DUBIOUS PROGNOSIS

The long-term prognosis of the first permanent molars needs to be considered at 8–9 years of age. If of dubious quality (*see* Plate 10) extraction and space closure makes a lot of sense. Since an important aim of dental care at this age is to engender dental health in adult life (including the avoidance of a continual need for replacement restorations), it is very wrong to attempt to conserve teeth avoidably and to saddle the patient with a restorative handicap for the rest of his or her days.

The extraction of poor first permanent molars at this time from crowded arches provides the best chance for the spontaneous resolution of crowding and the satisfactory eruption of the second permanent molars in contact with the second premolars, without excessive tipping (Fig. 14.1*a* and *b*, p. 98). The outcome following extraction at a later age depends on whether crowding has become concentrated in the premolar region following the previous loss of deciduous molars. When this has occurred, most of the extraction space can be occupied by the erupting premolars and a good result is obtained because the second permanent molars have very little residual space into which to tip mesially (Fig. 14.2*a* and *b*, p. 99).

Where the premolar region is not crowded, residual space closure is likely to be less complete and the contact points between the second permanent molars and second premolars will be less

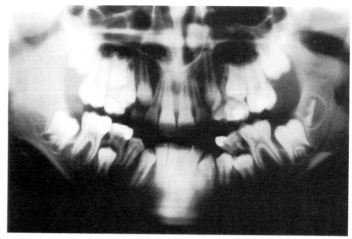

a

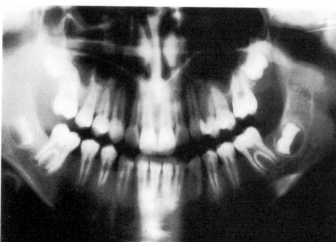

b

Fig. 14.1a and **b** *a = OPG showing dentition at 9 years of age prior to the extraction of the first permanent molars. Note that the root formation of the second permanent molars had not passed the bifurcation stage. b = OPG showing that satisfactory space closure has occurred at the extraction sites.*

satisfactory than if the extractions had been carried out earlier (Fig. 14.3*a* and *b*, p. 100).

The decision to extract all four first permanent molars is easier if all of these teeth are of poor prognosis. What does the clinician do, however, when this is not the case? The following are guiding principles.

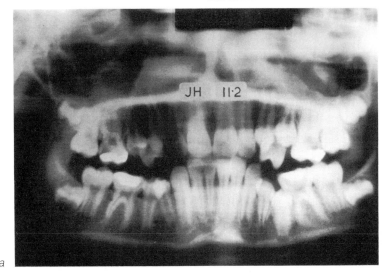

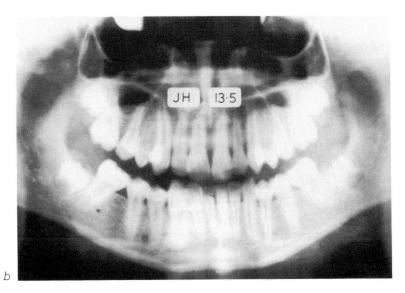

Fig. 14.2a and **b** a = OPG of a patient at 11 years and 2 months when root formation of the second permanent molars was very nearly complete. Many deciduous teeth had been extracted previously and the patient presented initially with considerable crowding in the premolar/canine regions. All four first permanent molars were extracted. b = OPG showing that satisfactory space closure has occurred.

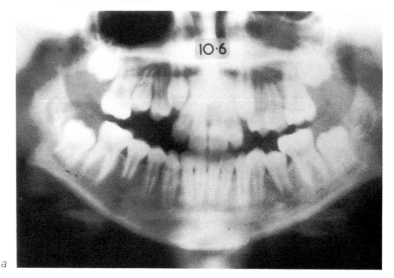

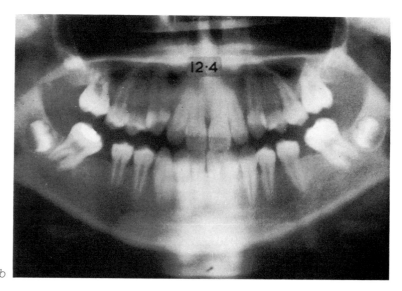

Fig. 14.3a and **b** a = OPG taken at 10 years and 6 months of age when root formation of the second permanent molars was well advanced in a patient with little or no premolar crowding. Nevertheless, all four first permanent molars were extracted. b = Two years later, excessive mesial tipping of second permanent molars has taken place and incomplete space closure will remain. This is a typical outcome under these circumstances.

A Maxillary First Permanent Molar with a Poor Prognosis and the Opposing First Permanent Molar with a Good Prognosis

Generally speaking, if a maxillary first permanent molar is to be extracted and the maxillary second molar is unerupted, then only this first molar need be removed. Unerupted maxillary second permanent molars are particularly good at moving mesially and erupting adjacent to the second premolar. An extraction this far posteriorly in the maxillary arch would have little effect on the centre-line and so there would be no need for a balancing extraction on the other side of the arch.

If the maxillary second permanent molar is in occlusion at the time the maxillary first molar is extracted, then the second molar would be hindered in its mesial migration on account of intercuspation with the opposing teeth unless the mandibular first permanent molar also is removed. It appears that buccal segments are better at coming mesially if opposing teeth can move forward together[3].

A Mandibular First Permanent Molar with a Poor Prognosis and the Opposing First Permanent Molar with a Good Prognosis

Where a mandibular first permanent molar has a poor prognosis, then it is wise to remove also the opposing maxillary first molar. This recommendation would apply irrespective of whether or not the mandibular second molar had erupted, because this latter tooth is not particularly good at moving mesially, and such movement can readily be prevented by an unopposed and over-erupted maxillary first permanent molar.

Unilateral Opposing First Permanent Molars with a Poor Prognosis

Where opposing first permanent molars on one side have a poor prognosis (or whenever both are to be extracted for the reasons mentioned above) and where those on the other side are to be retained, then it is wise to balance the extractions by removing also the second deciduous molars on this other side. This assumes that no extractions have already taken place in these contralateral quadrants and that there is labial segment crowding. Crowding will then resolve on the side where the permanent molars were removed and be transferred to the premolar region on the other side. This resulting premolar crowding can be treated by the extraction of the maxillary and mandibular first premolars on that side in due course.

Absent Third Molars

In patients with crowding, the absence of third molars should not affect the decision to extract poor quality first permanent molars.

Are There Situations When it Would be Better to Retain First Permanent Molars Even Though Their Prognosis is Dubious?

Where there is spacing in the arches, retention of all the permanent teeth is the only realistic way of maintaining the arches intact, so there is no gain in electively extracting restorable first permanent molars. Clearly it is also inappropriate to extract a first permanent molar in an arch with crowding if the adjacent second premolar is found to be developmentally absent unless, of course, the first permanent molar is totally unsavable.

Class II Division 1 Malocclusions

Present day thinking on the management of Class II division 1 patients, where the prognosis of the first permanent molars is poor and where there is crowding in both arches, is that extractions should be carried out at 8–9 years of age as for Class I patients[4]. These patients should then be reviewed when the second permanent molars, premolars and canines have erupted fully, and a decision made at that time on treatment to reduce the overjet.

Class II Division 2 Malocclusions

If fixed appliances are to be used eventually to correct maxillary incisor retroclination in Class II division 2 patients, it is not essential to remove poor prognosis first permanent molars in the mixed dentition unless symptoms make this a necessity. These extractions can be delayed until the second permanent molars have erupted fully. The production of good alignment between the second molars and second premolars can then be accomplished satisfactorily with fixed appliances at the same time as aligning the incisors.

Furthermore, where a traumatic overbite is causing damage to the periodontal tissues at the mixed dentition stage, the extraction of first permanent molars should be delayed, as a maxillary removable appliance will be needed to produce some overbite reduction, and such an appliance is best retained by the first permanent molars. The appliance should be worn until sufficient numbers of permanent teeth have erupted to permit orthodontic treatment to correct the incisor relationship.

Class III Malocclusions

Where incisor crossbites are to be corrected in the mixed dentition, the extraction of first permanent molars should be delayed until after the incisors have been aligned and the appliance has been discarded. This is because the two maxillary first permanent molars will be needed to retain the appliance, while the mandibulars are required for the molar capping (posterior bite planes) to occlude against.

As has been mentioned in Chapter 5 (p. 35), those Class III patients in whom all the maxillary permanent incisors are in crossbite should be referred for advice in the mixed dentition as regards the timing of orthodontic treatment. If the treatment is to be deferred until the permanent dentition proper (and fixed appliances used at that time), then it may be appropriate to postpone the extraction of first molars until then.

BALANCING AND COMPENSATING EXTRACTIONS

There are times when conservative measures either fail or are inappropriate and teeth have to be extracted. It is important to appreciate that the unilateral extraction of a deciduous molar or canine in a crowded dentition will localise the crowding to the extraction site. The first permanent molars will move mesially towards the extraction site, while the crowded incisors will move distally. The resulting occlusal asymmetry, with the incisors

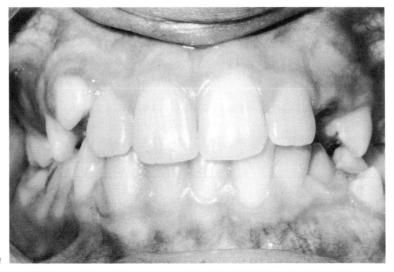

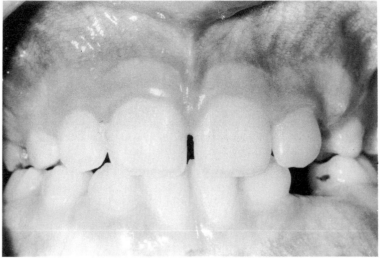

Fig. 14.4a and **b** a = Patient aged 11 years and 2 months with a Class I occlusion. The upper right deciduous canine and lower left deciduous first molar
had been lost 3 years previously. This has resolved the incisor crowding, but
at the expense of an upper centre-line shift to the right and a lower
centre-line shift to the left. b = By comparison, another patient (aged 9 years
3 months) with a Class I occlusion had previously lost the four deciduous
canines and the lower left first deciduous molar. Incisor crowding has been
resolved by symmetrical distal drift, with the result that centre-line shift has
not occurred.

taking on a centre-line discrepancy (Fig. 14.4*a* and *b*), will complicate any future orthodontic treatment. It is, therefore, often appropriate also to remove other teeth in the same or opposing arch as a preventive measure against the development of such an occlusal disturbance.

THE NEED FOR BALANCING EXTRACTIONS

The question is often asked as to whether this resulting asymmetry really matters, particularly as most patients do not notice a shift of the centre-line. The answer lies in the complexities it produces. Orthodontic treatment of patients with asymmetrical crowding is difficult. The extraction of all four first premolars is still usually necessary, and unless the occlusal asymmetries are corrected, excess residual space remains in those quadrants where early loss has not taken place (Fig. 14.5*a* and *b*, p. 106). These spaces would remain after treatment, as cuspal locks tend to maintain existing molar relationships[3].

In the situation described in Fig. 14.5*a* (p. 106) it would require a specialist to close the residual spaces and obtain a satisfactory Class I occlusion with correct molar relationships and correction of the centre-line discrepancy. Fixed appliances are nearly always necessary for the correction of these centre-line discrepancies.

There is no doubt that orthodontic treatment is simpler if the centre-lines coincide at the start of treatment, particularly if all the first premolars are to be extracted and removable appliances are to be used in the maxillary arch only. With the centre-lines coinciding and all the teeth in a Class I relationship, any remaining spaces at opposing extraction sites will be equal in extent (Fig. 14.5*b*, p. 106). When the appliance is finally discarded, the buccal segments are then able to move mesially together, thereby closing opposing spaces simultaneously.

It is abundantly clear that it is often good sense to balance the enforced extraction of deciduous molars and canines if the arches are crowded, in order to prevent displacement of the centre-lines (Fig. 14.4*b*)[1]. The balancing extraction is usually that of the contralateral tooth.

Balancing extractions are not required where:

● the dentition is spaced;
● a previous extraction in the same arch was balanced;

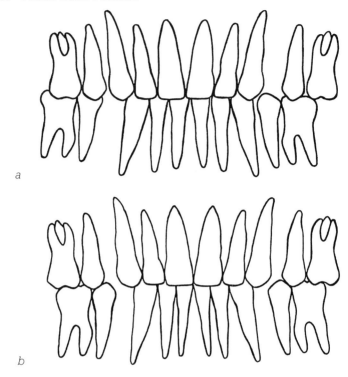

Fig. 14.5a and **b** a = *Diagrammatic representation of the occlusion following orthodontic treatment for a patient in which there had previously been early loss of a deciduous molar or canine in the upper right and lower left quadrants. All the first premolars had been extracted to resolve the crowding, but no steps had been taken to correct the centre-line discrepancy nor the dissimilar molar relationships. Excess residual space, therefore, remains in the upper left and lower right quadrants. b = The desired occlusion at the end of orthodontic treatment if residual extraction spaces are to have a chance of closing spontaneously through mesial drift of the buccal segments. The canine occlusion should match the molar occlusion so that opposing spaces are equal in extent.*

- the tooth requiring enforced extraction is close to exfoliation

COMPENSATING EXTRACTIONS

A compensating extraction is when the corresponding tooth in the opposing quadrant is also removed. The effect of these extractions is to maintain the existing molar occlusion, so that opposing buccal segments can then move mesially together.

Compensating extractions of permanent teeth are desirable (even essential) where there is crowding in both arches; they help ensure satisfactory space closure at the extraction sites. The need for compensating deciduous extractions is more debatable.

When second deciduous molars are shed naturally, then the occlusion of the first permanent molars typically alters from being a half unit Class II to become Class I (Fig. 14.6*a*, p. 108)[5]. The same change in molar occlusion would occur if a mandibular second deciduous molar, say, is removed without a compensating extraction being carried out in the opposing arch (Fig. 14.6*b*, p. 108). However, the molar occlusion would become more Class II in those situations where a maxillary second deciduous molar is removed without compensating (Fig. 14.6*c*, p. 108).

When resolving crowding in both arches and producing a Class I incisor relationship, one permanent tooth (often a first pre-molar), is usually extracted from each quadrant. It is obviously helpful if the buccal occlusion at the start of treatment is Class I, for the molar occlusion at the end of treatment would also have to be Class I if all residual spaces are to be closed. Thus, in certain situations, compensating extractions of deciduous molars or canines can simplify future orthodontic treatment by preventing the molar occlusion from becoming Class II.

Enforced Extraction of a Mandibular Deciduous Molar or Canine

Usually there is no need to carry out a compensating extraction when a mandibular deciduous molar or canine has to be lost, as in most cases the molar occlusion merely becomes more Class I as a result of mesial movement of the mandibular first permanent molars. Providing the mandibular arch is not spaced, then only a balancing extraction need be considered for these patients.

Enforced Extraction of a Maxillary Deciduous Molar or Canine

In addition to balancing, there are reasonable grounds for com-pensating the enforced extraction of a maxillary deciduous molar

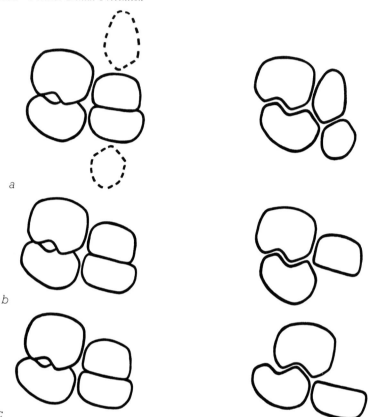

Fig. 14.6a, b and **c** a = *Following the exfoliation of second deciduous molars, a half unit Class II occlusion of the first permanent molars can be expected to become Class I because of the greater amount of leeway space to be taken up in the lower arch. b = However, following the extraction of a mandibular deciduous molar or canine, the first permanent molar in the quadrant concerned would move mesially, thereby changing a half unit Class II molar occlusion into a Class I relationship. c = Following the extraction of a maxillary deciduous molar or canine, there would be a tendency for the first permanent molar in the quadrant concerned to move mesially. Unless a compensating extraction is also carried out, a half unit Class II molar occlusion would become more Class II.*

or canine where there is crowding in both arches and where the occlusion of the first permanent molars is a half unit Class II. The reader will appreciate that the balancing extraction would itself need to be similarly compensated (thus four teeth would be extracted).

These extractions can be expected to prevent the molar occlusion from becoming more Class II. It should be pointed out, however, that this is not too critical, for if compensating extractions are not done, then the correction of the resulting Class II molar occlusion would not be a difficult procedure to carry out and can be accomplished with a maxillary removable appliance and extra-oral anchorage. The relatively straightforward nature of such an appliance system should be contrasted with the fixed appliances which are often necessary to restore arch symmetry if balancing extractions are omitted. The critical point to note is that it is much more important to balance the extraction of deciduous molars and canines than to compensate.

Developmentally Absent Permanent Teeth

The compensating extraction of a deciduous tooth should be considered when there is developmental absence of the permanent successor, subject to assessment by a specialist at the early mixed dentition stage. If a mandibular second premolar, for example, is developmentally absent and the arches are crowded, then the extraction of the two second deciduous molars on that side may be advised in order to encourage resolution of the crowding and mesial movement of the molars. The maxillary second premolar can then be removed later when it erupts.

THE MANAGEMENT OF SUBMERGING DECIDUOUS MOLARS

Submerging deciduous molars have no functional use and can lead to food packing and plaque accumulation. If there is no permanent successor then the submerging tooth should be removed.

If the permanent successor is present then extraction of the submerging tooth, with 'balancing' if necessary, should be carried out if it has submerged to the extent that any further submergence would make extraction difficult or if eruption of the permanent tooth is becoming hindered.

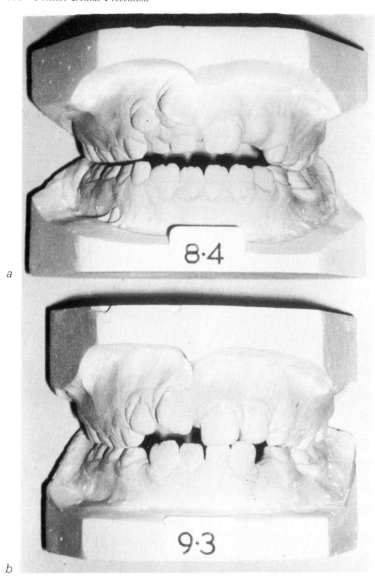

a

b

Fig. 14.7a, *b* and *c* *a and b = The extraction of the upper right deciduous incisors has allowed the ectopically erupting permanent incisors to improve their position spontaneously. c = In another patient (7 years old), the lower lateral incisors are erupting lingually. The deciduous lateral incisors are firm. These and the deciduous canines should be removed in order to permit the lower lateral incisors to align spontaneously.*

THE MANAGEMENT OF IMPACTED FIRST PERMANENT MOLARS

Occasionally a first permanent molar (usually maxillary) becomes impacted against the second deciduous molar and fails to erupt fully. Treatments variously described include: moving the first permanent molar distally by orthodontic means, disimpacting the first permanent molar by means of brass wire tightened around its mesial contact point[6] or discing the distal surface of the second deciduous molar. The problem with any prolonged procedure is that the time involved will usually encroach upon the 2 years or so of goodwill that most patients are prepared to give to orthodontic treatment. In many cases, it is wise to take the easy route and extract the second deciduous molar and deal with the resulting premolar crowding when the first premolars have erupted.

THE MANAGEMENT OF OTHER ECTOPICALLY ERUPTING PERMANENT TEETH

Where a premolar or permanent incisor erupts slightly ectopically, the roots of the deciduous predecessor often do not resorb uniformly and the successor is deflected even further off course. These deciduous teeth should be removed (Fig. 14.7*a*).

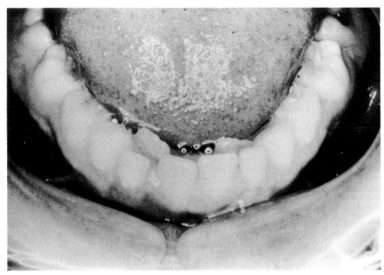

c

Permanent mandibular incisors can sometimes erupt lingual to the deciduous incisors so that the appearance is of a double row of teeth. If a single tooth is involved and the associated deciduous tooth is close to exfoliation, then nothing further need be done. However, at the other extreme, several permanent incisors may be affected and the deciduous teeth remain firm (Fig. 14.7c, p. 111). The deciduous mandibular incisors and canines should then be extracted in order to permit the tongue to push the crowns of the permanent incisors labially into their intended positions.

The roots of non-vital deciduous teeth frequently do not resorb easily and the erupting permanent tooth risks becoming deflected. If this is the case, then the deciduous tooth should be removed.

SUMMARY

1. Always refer a patient for specialist advice if serial extractions are contemplated.
2. The long-term prognosis of the first permanent molars must be assessed at 8 or 9 years of age. If the prognosis of these teeth is poor and the dentition is not spaced, then their removal at this time should be considered.
3. The enforced extraction of deciduous molars and canines should be balanced in patients where the dentition is well aligned or crowded (i.e. not spaced), in order to prevent lateral displacement of the centre-line.
4. Where the buccal segments are in a half unit Class II relationship and a maxillary deciduous molar or canine is to be lost, then a compensating extraction is desirable to prevent the buccal occlusion from becoming more Class II.

REFERENCES

1. Foster T. D. (1982). *A Textbook of Orthodontics*, 2nd Ed., pp. 224–8. Oxford: Blackwell Scientific Publications.
2. Mills J. R. E. (1982). *Principles and Practice of Orthodontics*. pp. 105–6. Edinburgh: Churchill Livingstone.
3. Stephens C. D., Lloyd T. G. (1980). Changes in molar occlusion after extraction of all first premolars: a follow-up study of Class II division 1 cases treated with removable appliances. *Brit. J. Orthod*; **7**: 139–44.

4. Houston W. J. B. (1976). *Walther's Orthodontic Notes*, 3rd Ed. p. 83. Bristol: John Wright and Sons.
5. Carlsen D. B., Meredith H. V. (1960). Biologic variation in selected relationships of opposing posterior teeth. *Angle Orthod*; **30**: 162–73.
6. Andlaw R. J., Rock W. P. (1982). *A Manual of Paedodontics*. pp. 126–7. Edinburgh: Churchill Livingstone.

15

The Control of Class II Division 1 Malocclusion with Myofunctional Appliances

C. D. STEPHENS

With greater emphasis now being placed on the role of the general dentist in the management of the developing occlusion, it is appropriate to consider the present place which myofunctional appliances occupy in interceptive orthodontics. The past 10 years have seen a great revival of interest in the use of these appliances both in the UK and in the USA. What are myofunctional appliances and what contribution can they make to dental health in adult life through the early treatment of malocclusion?

There are two broad categories of myofunctional appliance:

- those which are primarily rigid and are essentially a maxillary and mandibular base plate joined together (Fig. 15.1). Most of these have their origins in the Andresen appliance;
- those which are more flexible, incorporating a much greater amount of wire work, of which the best known is the Frankel Function Regulator. These are more complex in construction, adjustment and use, and are outside the scope of the non-specialist.

The discussion below is confined to the principles and use of appliances in the first group, of which there are very many examples[1].

Although myofunctional appliances are described which may be effective in the treatment of Class I and Class III malocclusion, it is in the treatment of Class II division 1 malocclusion in the late mixed dentition that myofunctional appliances enjoy greatest popularity. By and large they produce gross changes in arch relationships, there being very little capacity for them to achieve

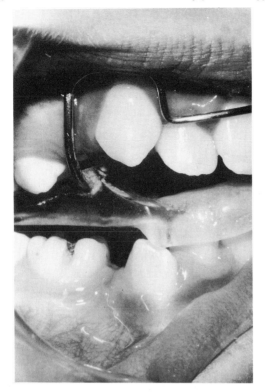

Fig. 15.1 *A Harvold Activator in use following premolar extractions.*

intra-arch tooth movement. If tooth alignment within an arch is required, this must be done later with removable or fixed appliances when the permanent dentition has erupted. Exaggerated claims have been made by enthusiastic advocates claiming significant advantages of a particular type of myofunctional appliance, but the evidence so far produced suggests that the clinical effect achieved by all varieties is very similar.

The precise mode of action of functional appliances is not fully understood, but it clearly involves forces derived from the muscles of mastication and perhaps also those of facial expression. There is, however, general agreement that myofunctional appliances are most effective when used during periods of rapid facial growth[2,3]. In such circumstances they achieve their effect in the treatment of Class II malocclusion by inducing one or more of the following changes:

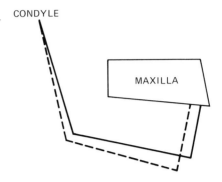

Fig. 15.2 *Diagram showing (hatched line) how the skeletal discrepancy is accentuated in the anteroposterior plane as a result of increased lower face height following wearing a myofunctional appliance.*

- a reduction in the forward development of the maxilla— this is sometimes known as the 'headgear effect';
- an alteration in the pattern of mandibular development— either the rate of growth, the total amount of growth, or the direction of growth;
- a forward relocation of the glenoid fossa—with consequent forward positioning of the mandible;
- dentoalveolar changes—both by tipping of the anterior teeth and by eruption and mesial migration of the posterior teeth. This is generally agreed to be the major therapeutic effect[4].

Careful cephalometric assessment should be made before commencing myofunctional appliance therapy, for these appliances cause the molars to erupt further than would otherwise be the case, thereby increasing the lower face height. Particularly, where the pattern of growth is already rather vertical (determined by the cephalometric analysis), this can be a great disadvantage, for it has the effect of accentuating the skeletal discrepancy in the anteroposterior plane (Fig. 15.2).

THE RELEVANCE OF GROWTH IN FUNCTIONAL APPLIANCE TREATMENT

With conventional orthodontic appliances growth in general may be desirable, for example, in the reduction of an excessive incisor overbite through an increase in the lower face height. However, with functional appliances, growth is essential, since without alveolar and mandibular growth, the appliance can achieve no more than conventional orthodontic tooth movement[4]. In patients who exhibit rapid and favourable facial growth during the period when they are wearing a functional appliance, sagittal changes occur with remarkable rapidity. On the other hand, if the patient is undergoing little or no facial growth, treatment changes are so small that the clinician may suspect that the patient is failing to wear the appliance satisfactorily. It is, therefore, important to make some attempt to monitor growth. One of the easiest ways is to record the patient's height at each visit during treatment.

Because myofunctional appliances produce gross changes in arch relationship and are unable to produce individual tooth movement, their use was originally confined to patients in whom there was no crowding (i.e. where extractions are not required). It has, however, been appreciated for some time that the Andresen appliance can be used very effectively to treat patients with Class II division 1 malocclusions in which there has been early removal of all four first permanent molars[5]. Unfortunately the design of this appliance limits spontaneous tooth movement, where, for example, it is still desirable for the second molars to move mesially. Fortunately, the advent of the Harvold Activator (which does not have extensions of the acrylic to engage the lingual embrasure areas and lock the teeth) has made it possible to carry out functional appliance treatment without difficulty during the late mixed dentition. It is even possible to extract first premolars while the activator is being worn and take advantage of spontaneous alignment prior to the fitting of conventional fixed or removable appliances[6].

THE USE OF MYOFUNCTIONAL APPLIANCES IN PREVENTION

Apart from exceptional cases, the child of 7–10 years is not likely to be sufficiently mature to cope with wearing a bulky myofunctional appliance. There also appears to be a limit to the total amount of cooperation that is available, and 3 years of appliance wear seems to be about this limit for most patients. As orthodontic treatment cannot be completed until the permanent dentition is established, it is usual to delay the start of treatment until the patient is aged around 11 years, except where there are obvious advantages. Three situations in which early treatment with myofunctional appliances may be beneficial are:

- The early treatment of prominent incisors in an endeavour to reduce the risk of accidental trauma;
- the early treatment of severe skeletal Class II division 1 malocclusion where the additional effect of early treatment may enable surgical correction to be avoided and a highly satisfactory result be obtained by orthodontic means alone;
- the early treatment of Class II division 2 malocclusion.

Early Treatment of Prominent Incisors

The definitive treatment of most malocclusions must await the eruption of premolar and canine teeth. This is because decisions about extractions cannot be made reliably until this time (and even where they can, few dentists would feel justified in carrying out surgical removal of unerupted teeth). In most instances this delay is of advantage since the eruption of premolar teeth coincides with the growth spurt and enables treatment to be accomplished rapidly. However, the clinician will frequently be under some pressure to institute early orthodontic treatment from parents of children with Class II division 1 malocclusions. In general, such pressure should be firmly resisted.

In weighing up the pros and cons of interventive orthodontics when there is a severe overjet, the lifetime's potential consequences of trauma should be considered. A damaged incisor can so easily enter a repeat restorative cycle whereby a series of composite restorations is replaced by a series of crowns, endodontic treatments, post-crowns, repairs of lateral root perforations, bridges, etc. It must be remembered that almost one-half of 12-year-old children who have an overjet of 7 mm or more (about 9% of the child population) have suffered accidental damage to one or more of their maxillary incisor teeth[7]. Such damage would seem to be particularly likely where the lips are grossly incompetent.

If appliance therapy is commenced early, it should not last too long (e.g. 9–12 months). A functional appliance can then be worn at night to maintain the improved occlusion, and patients seem to accept this. Just worn at night, the functional appliance cannot, of course, be expected to achieve tooth movement *per se*. This plan of action should be considered for those patients with severely increased overjets who are at particular risk from direct trauma.

Early Treatment for the Severe Skeletal II Malocclusion

It is now appreciated that myofunctional appliances are particularly appropriate in the early treatment of the very severe Class II malocclusion for which surgery appears to be unavoidable. In a significant proportion of these patients a combination of favourable growth and enthusiastic wear can produce remarkable effects, sufficient to obviate the need for surgical correction in the late teens (Fig. 15.3*a* and *b*, p. 120). It will be appreciated, of course, that myofunctional treatment is seldom so effective as to fully reduce a severe incisor overjet, but it can at least bring the malocclusion within the range of conventional fixed appliance treatment. It is not appropriate for the general practitioner to treat these patients, though he or she does have an essential role to play in their early recognition and referral to a specialist centre for a combined orthodontic and surgical opinion.

Early Treatment of Class II Division 2 Incisor Relationships

Where there is a traumatic incisor overbite in a patient with a Class II division 2 malocclusion it is sometimes appropriate to procline the maxillary incisors with a conventional orthodontic appliance (to achieve a Class II division 1 malocclusion) and then to use a myofunctional appliance to reduce the overjet. This type of functional appliance has to be carefully designed to avoid the incisors returning to their pretreatment relationship.

LIMITATIONS

Myofunctional appliances, in common with all orthodontic appliances, are only effective if worn conscientiously. Although there is no necessity for full time wear, 14–16 h of wear each day is normally desirable. Because these appliances are bulky, they tend to be difficult to get used to and sadly many patients fail to come to terms with them. For example, myofunctional appliances may not

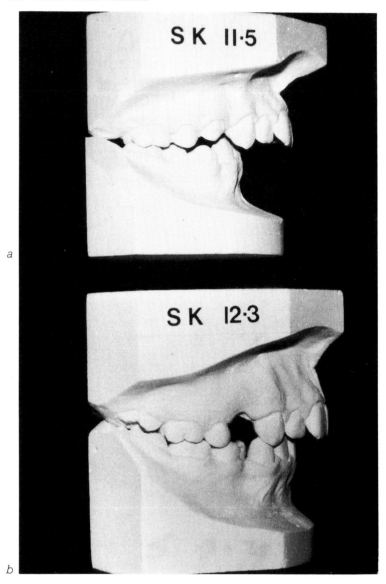

Fig. 15.3a and **b** *Study models of a patient with a severe Class II malocclusion. a = Before treatment; b = After treatment with a myofunctional appliance. The next stage of the treatment required a fixed appliance.*

be tolerated for patients who mouth-breathe. Prior assessment of patient cooperation is, therefore, crucial to success. Studies have shown that if marked progress (at least 4 mm of overjet reduction) has not been achieved during the first 6 months of wear, there is little likelihood of treatment being successfully concluded and an alternative method of treatment should be employed.

It is conceivable that myofunctional appliances may have a role in the treatment of handicapped patients, although as yet no studies exist which report their use. They are very resistant to accidental damage, and because of their loose fit, some orthodontists consider that they promote salivation and may therefore be of positive advantage in terms of reducing caries progression.

REFERENCES

1. Graber T. M., Neumann B. (1977). *Removable Orthodontic Appliances*, 2nd Ed. Philadelphia: W. B. Saunders Company.
2. Ahlgren J., Laurin C. (1976). Late results of activator treatment: a cephalometric study. *Brit. J. Orthod*; **3**: 181–7.
3. McNamara J. A. (1984). Dentofacial adaptions in adult patients following functional regulator therapy. *Amer. J. Orthod*; **3**: 57–71.
4. Mills J. R. E. (1978). The effect of orthodontic treatment on the skeletal pattern. *Brit. J. Orthod*; **5**: 133–43.
5. Tulley W. J., Campbell A. (1970). *A Manual of Practical Orthodontics*. Bristol: John Wright.
6. Pfeiffer J. P., Grobety D. (1982). A philosophy of combined orthopaedic orthodontic treatment. *Amer. J. Orthod*; **81**: 185–201.
7. Todd J. E., Dodd T. (1985). *Children's dental health in the United Kingdom 1983*. p. 100. London: HMSO.

16

Prevention and the Avulsed Anterior Tooth

R. J. ANDLAW and C. D. STEPHENS

PREVENTION

About a quarter of the children in the UK suffer trauma to their anterior teeth by the age of 15 years (*see* Chapter 1, p. 3)[1]. Much of this cannot be prevented, but injuries to teeth caused while playing contact sports can be significantly reduced by the wearing of mouth-guards. These should certainly be recommended for children involved in the rougher sports (e.g. rugby football) and particularly for the child with an increased overjet and incompetent lips, whose teeth are especially at risk[1]. It should, however, be appreciated that trauma during sport only accounts for perhaps 10% of injuries to teeth in children. Playground and bicycle accidents are much more common causes.

The most satisfactory mouthguards are those made on a plaster/stone model of the patient's maxillary arch. The material most commonly used is polyvinyl acetate-polyethylene. A sheet of the material 3 mm or 4 mm thick is moulded to the model; usually this is done in an apparatus that heats the material and moulds it under either pressure or vacuum, but it can be done by heating the material in hot water and moulding by hand. The plastic is then cut to the shape shown in Fig. 16.1. Buccally and labially the periphery should be about 3 mm short of the muco-buccal fold, and palatally it should be about 10 mm from the molar gingival margins and behind the rugae. Distally the mouthguard need only extend as far as the first permanent molars. The periphery is smoothed by passing it over a flame.

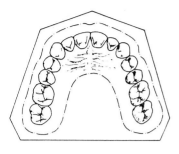 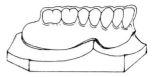

Fig. 16.1 *Polyvinyl acetate-polyethylene mouthguard on a study model.* (Reproduced by kind permission of Churchill Livingstone, publishers of *A Manual of Paedodontics.*)

Mouthguards made as described above are very satisfactory because they fit closely; they are, however, moderately expensive because surgery and laboratory work are required. Other types of mouthguards may be purchased relatively cheaply and moulded by the patient in his or her own mouth, but these are often ill-fitting and therefore tend to be less satisfactory[2].

TRAUMATIC LOSS OF A CENTRAL INCISOR

The traumatic loss of a central incisor is extremely distressing to both the child and to the accompanying parent, and the question arises: what are the implications of the loss of the tooth on long-term dental health and status? Clearly, an orthodontic assessment is required. However, under the circumstances of having just lost a tooth, detailed examination of the occlusion cannot be undertaken even if the patient is at a suitable age at which orthodontic treatment could confidently be planned. Nor can the various implications of emergency treatment be discussed adequately at this time. Any orthodontic treatment plan must be preceded by a thorough clinical examination to allow an assessment of all the aetiological factors that may be present. It is also common practice to discuss the various treatment options with the patient and parent and, if necessary, allow them adequate time to go away and think these over before making a commitment to long-term treatment which may involve considerable cooperation on their part.

Thus, decisions which may profoundly affect the occlusion cannot and should not be made hurriedly on the occasion that a child presents with a lost tooth. Therefore, in order to avoid reducing later treatment options, *initial treatment should always be directed towards maintaining the incisor space*—be this by implanting the original tooth or by using some form of temporary space maintainer. Failure to do this will generally result in any occlusal problem becoming unnecessarily complicated, sometimes to the point where even complex treatment cannot fully resolve matters (Fig. 16.2*a* and *b*). Occasionally space will be preserved unnecessarily in the short-term. But these occasions are few and far between.

It should be remembered that in the growing child, particularly where adjacent teeth have recently erupted, a central incisor space will close extremely rapidly. In a week up to 2 mm can be lost, and therefore treatment to achieve space maintenance should be carried out immediately. Where the tooth is not replanted and a laboratory is on site, an immediate denture should be made. This should be clasped, since 'spoon' dentures do not reliably maintain space (as the denture tooth is free to be gradually displaced occlusally as adjacent teeth encroach). It is also a wise precaution to include well-retained wire spurs mesially and distally to the denture tooth so that space maintenance will continue even if the tooth becomes fractured from the baseplate. If circumstances do not permit the fitting of a denture on the day of the accident, some other form of temporary space maintenance (e.g. cold curing acrylic resin, wire bonded to adjacent teeth using the acid etch technique) must be employed until it can be provided. Subsequently, when the patient is happy with his or her restored appearance, radiographs and study models can be obtained and the nature and timing of subsequent treatment can be considered, seeking consultant advice as necessary.

REPLANTATION OF AN AVULSED TOOTH

Replantation of an avulsed permanent tooth is usually justified, especially in children, despite the fact that the long-term prognosis is generally poor. One of the most important factors determining the prognosis is the length of time that the tooth remains out of the mouth. Therefore, if a parent telephones to report the accident, he or she should be encouraged to replant the tooth. Instructions should be given: to hold the tooth by its crown, not by its

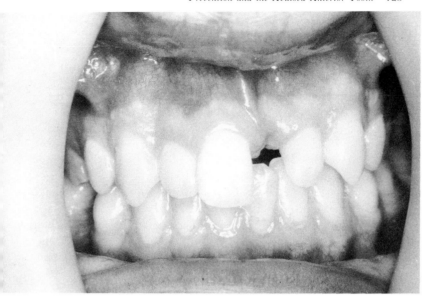

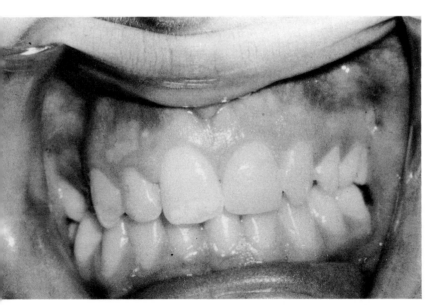

Fig. 16.2a and **b** *Failure to maintain the space after loss of the upper left central incisor has left these two patients and their dentists with complex problems.*

root; to remove any particles of dirt that may be present on the root surface very gently with a moist tissue (moistened preferably with saliva rather than with water); to replant the tooth carefully in its socket; to ask the child to keep it in place by biting on a handkerchief; and to report to the surgery as quickly as possible.

If the parent is unwilling or unable to carry out these instructions, directions must be given on how best to transport the tooth to the surgery; this is a crucial factor influencing the prognosis, because it is essential to maintain the vitality of the periodontal tissues attached to the root surface. The ideal method is for the tooth to be placed in the child's mouth (or even the parent's mouth); the lower labial sulcus may be recommended as a safe place. If they are unwilling to do this they should be advised to place the tooth in milk, which has been shown to be a satisfactory medium for maintaining the vitality of the periodontal tissues[3]; water is a poor medium. If milk is not available, the tooth should be placed in a clean tissue or handkerchief moistened with the child's or the parent's saliva.

When the patient reaches the surgery, the tooth should immediately be placed in saline so that it can be examined and cleaned. A dental and medical history is taken and the extra-oral and intra-oral injuries are examined. If it is decided to replant the tooth, this should be done without further delay; the taking of radiographs may be postponed until after the tooth has been replanted (except when there is a suspicion of alveolar fracture that would complicate replantation). The periodontal tissues adhering to the root surface should be cleaned if necessary by dabbing gently with gauze soaked in saline, but great care must be taken to avoid damaging them. Local analgesia may not be required to replant the tooth but would, of course, be required before suturing soft tissue lacerations.

The replanted tooth must be splinted. If the tooth is in contact with adjacent teeth, the incisal half of the labial surfaces of the replanted tooth and of at least one tooth mesial and distal to it should be etched (most conveniently with a gel preparation) and a layer of epimine resin ('Scutan') or of acrylic resin ('Trim') flowed over the etched area (Fig. 16.3). If there are spaces between the teeth, a piece of orthodontic wire (or even a paper clip) may be adapted to the labial surfaces of the teeth and attached with epimine or acrylic resin. These resins are preferred to composite resin for splint construction because they are adequately

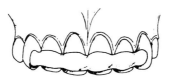

Fig. 16.3 *Acid etch-retained epimine or acrylic resin splint to stabilise a loosened or replanted tooth.* (Reproduced by kind permission of Churchill Livingstone, publishers of *A Manual of Paedodontics.*)

retained on acid-etched enamel, yet relatively easy to remove at the end of the splinting period.

Where splinting to adjacent teeth is not possible (e.g. in a young child with lateral incisors only partially erupted), a different kind of splint is required. A suitable splint may be made on a model of the patient's dentition. An alginate impression is taken, supporting the replanted tooth with a suitably bent piece of wire or dental instrument, as shown in Fig. 16.4 (p. 128). An acrylic splint may be made, overlapping the incisal edges of the incisors and incorporating Adams cribs for retention (Fig. 16.5, p. 128)[4]. Alternatively, a mouthguard may be made as described above (p. 122). Unless the splint can be made on the same day, a temporary splint is required, e.g. zinc oxide–eugenol within thin metal foil, or an adhesive 'bandage' ('Stomahesive').

The acrylic splint or the mouthguard is used as a removable splint, but the patient should be instructed to wear it continuously for the first 3 days; thereafter it should be removed after meals for cleaning and for toothbrushing. Removable splints may be used for all splinting purposes, but the resin splints described above are generally preferred.

A course of antibiotics should be prescribed and arrangements should be made for a tetanus 'booster' injection to be given if the wound is contaminated and if the patient has not received tetanus immunisation within the previous 5 years.

The patient should be seen again after 1–2 weeks and the splint removed; longer splinting periods encourage ankylosis[5]. The tooth will not yet be firm in its socket and the patient must be advised to take sensible precautions.

Pulp death will almost inevitably occur, and root canal treatment should therefore be carried out as soon as possible. The only exception to this rule is when an immature tooth with a wide open root apex (e.g. in an 8 or 9-year-old child) is replanted within 2 h,

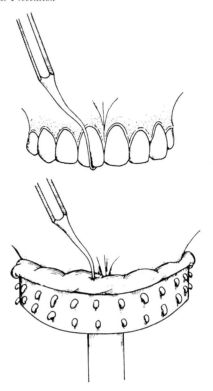

Fig. 16.4 *Supporting a replanted tooth with a modified dental instrument while taking an impression for a splint.* (Reproduced by kind permission of Churchill Livingstone, publishers of *A Manual of Paedodontics.*)

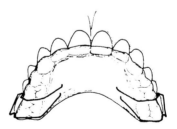

Fig. 16.5 *A removable acrylic splint to support a loosened or replanted tooth.* (Reproduced by kind permission of Churchill Livingstone, publishers of *A Manual of Paedodontics.*)

after having been kept moist with saliva or milk. In such a case it would be justifiable to keep the tooth under close clinical and radiographic review (about every month), and to carry out root canal treatment only if radiographic evidence of root resorption was noted. Root canal treatment in all cases should involve pulpectomy, reaming and filing of the canal, and filling with a calcium hydroxide paste. This procedure may possibly prevent or arrest root resorption. If root resorption is progressing rapidly, the calcium hydroxide should be replaced at about 2-monthly intervals in an attempt to control it. The canal should not be filled with a permanent material until there is radiographic evidence that no root resorption is occurring, or that it has been arrested.

For more detailed information on these procedures the reader is referred to Andreasen's authoritative text[6].

LONGER TERM TREATMENT OPTIONS

Where a tooth has been lost or where the prognosis for a replanted tooth is judged to be poor, there are two possibilities:

- maintaining the space for later prosthetic replacement;
- closing the space, either actively by means of an orthodontic appliance, or passively by 'mesial drift'.

With the patient who presents with an uncrowded Class I dentition (usually at the common age of injury this means a well aligned mandibular labial segment and a spaced maxillary labial segment) space cannot easily be closed and there is usually no alternative but to maintain it. However, most dentitions in the UK have some crowding, and traumatic injury is frequently associated with an increased incisor overjet which will later require reduction. Here it may appear attractive to use the space provided by the lost maxillary anterior tooth to relieve the crowding or to permit the overjet to be reduced. However, even in these circumstances, and certainly when it is a maxillary central incisor that has been lost, it is usually preferable to replace the tooth prosthetically, even when this means extracting sound premolar teeth later to permit the overjet to be reduced. This is because the alternative involves crowning or building up a lateral incisor so that it simulates the lost central. Such attempts are seldom completely successful, either in terms of appearance or in terms of the long-term health of the crowned lateral. Even where the lateral incisor is large and fixed appliance therapy has ensured that it is in an upright position in the middle of the space and a good crown (or composite crown) has been constructed, the aesthetic problem remains. On one side of the mouth the central incisor will be flanked by the smaller lateral; on the other, the crowned lateral will be next to a canine. The attractiveness of the final result rests to a very large extent on the shape and size of the canine. Where this is rather small and of a tapering form, a good result can sometimes be achieved. Otherwise, the appearance ranges from poor to unacceptable.

It is unusual for both upper central incisors to be avulsed, but if they are, initial prosthetic replacement is still the appropriate treatment. Just occasionally, space closure provides an acceptable solution where there is crowding.

OCCLUSION WITH THE MANDIBULAR ARCH

Having so far considered the problem purely in terms of the maxillary arch, it is important to remember that orthodontic treatment planning always begins in the lower arch. This is because the perimeter of the latter is determined by the soft tissues of the tongue, lips and cheeks and hence the labio-lingual positions of the lower teeth, unlike those in the maxillary arch, cannot be altered. The maxillary teeth have to be adapted to fit around the mandibular. It is helpful, perhaps, to reflect on the effect of the loss of a maxillary anterior tooth on the occlusion as a whole.

One of the aims of any orthodontic treatment plan should be to ensure that the patient achieves a well intercuspated occlusion. If the missing central incisor is replaced prosthetically, this objective will present no more occlusal problems than that of the original malocclusion. Thus, where dental crowding must be relieved, conventional symmetrical orthodontic extractions can be performed. It will also be appreciated that if a maxillary lateral incisor has been crowned to simulate a missing central incisor, the effect in terms of space is the same as if the lateral incisor had been removed (since the lateral now occupies the same amount of space as the central incisor once did). Assuming there is to be no residual space at the end of treatment, the maxillary canine will need to occlude with the mandibular canine and the lateral incisor. However, because of its greater labio-palatal dimension, it tends to stand rather proud of the arch, thereby emphasising its bulk. More importantly, in this position lateral excursions cannot take place freely and lateral stresses are placed upon the

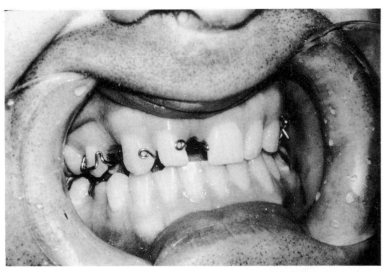

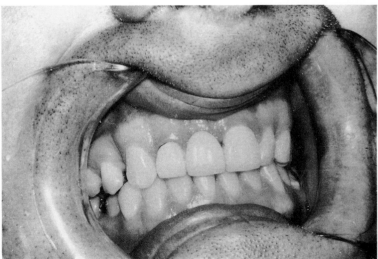

Fig. 16.6a and **b** *Removal of the maxillary right first premolar and orthodontic treatment (a) to create sufficient space for the prosthetic replacement of the missing central incisor (b).*

diminutive mandibular lateral incisor rather than upon the mandibular canine. Not infrequently it will later be decided, for both fuction and aesthetic purposes, to extract a premolar to permit the central incisor to be replaced prosthetically (Fig. 16.6*a* and *b*, p. 131).

REFERENCES

1. O'Mullane D. M. (1973). Some factors predisposing to injuries of permanent incisors in school children. *Brit. Dent. J*; **134**: 328–32.
2. Turner C. H. (1977). Mouth protectors. *Brit. Dent. J*; **143**: 82–6.
3. Blomlöf L., Otteskog P. (1980). Vitality of human periodontal ligament cells after storage in milk or saliva. *Scand. J. Dent. Res*; **88**: 436–40.
4. Andlaw R. J., Rock W. P. (1982). *A Manual of Paedodontics*. Edinburgh: Churchill Livingstone.
5. Andreasen J. O. (1975). The effect of splinting upon periodontal healing after replantation of permanent incisors in monkeys. *Acta Odont. Scand*; **33**: 313–23.
6. Andreasen J. O. (1981). *Traumatic Injuries of the Teeth*, 2nd Ed. Copenhagen: Munksgaard.

17

Prevention of Malocclusion after Eruption of the Second Permanent Molars

C. D. STEPHENS

There is a tendency for the perimeter of the dental arch to decrease in late childhood and early adult life[1], and this may lead to late crowding in the dental arches. If the dentist understands both the mechanisms involved and their management, he or she is in a position to interact, as necessary, in providing treatment, referring the patient, or providing informed reassurance.

In the ideal developing occlusion, the mesial migration initially produces closure of any spaces remaining within the dental arches at the end of the mixed dentition stage. Typically, these spaces are the remains of the physiological diastema in the upper arch and leeway space (excess space provided when the lower deciduous molars are shed) in the lower. In a crowded or potentially crowded dentition, no such space is or will be available and these growth-related changes are accompanied instead by the appearance of frank crowding.

It is principally the alignment of anterior teeth of the mandibular arch which is affected by these changes[2]. The appearance of lower incisor imbrication in young men between 14 and 18 years of age is so common that it is generally regarded as the norm. Similar crowding changes in girls are less obvious, perhaps because facial growth takes place about 2 years earlier, at a time when most of the increase in crowding is obscured by the change from the late mixed to permanent dentitions.

A small number of women complain of maxillary incisor imbrication in their late 20s and early 30s. At one time there was a tendency to blame periodontal disease as the cause. However, these changes can take place where bone support is normal, although they are more rapid and more marked where there is evidence of bone loss.

SIGNIFICANCE OF LATE CROWDING

There is no evidence that incisor imbrication is incompatible with dental health. Indeed, the endemically crowded British mandibular labial segment is generally the most lasting area of the dentition[3].

In the early stages of this imbrication process, there is unlikely to be an aesthetic problem. Few patients show much of their mandibular anterior teeth and even where they do, the crowding needs to be quite marked before it is obvious to the world. Nevertheless it is important to bear in mind that unless there is no occlusal contact between the maxillary and mandibular anterior teeth, irregularity in the lower arch will eventually be reflected in the alignment of the upper incisors. This is particularly so where there is a Class II division 2 incisor relationship. Here a crowded mandibular incisor will not only tend to carry a maxillary incisor labially, but it may itself be intruded (pushed apically) by resistance from the cingulum of its opposing tooth.

CONTRIBUTORY CAUSES OF LATE CROWDING

These may be considered as three-fold:

- posterior teeth moving anteriorly;
- the crowns of the mandibular anterior teeth moving lingually;
- narrowing of the mandibular arch.

Posterior Teeth Moving Anteriorly

Perhaps, not suprisingly, many of the factors which have been put forward as playing a part in the causation of late crowding are the same as those which are believed to be responsible for mesial drift.

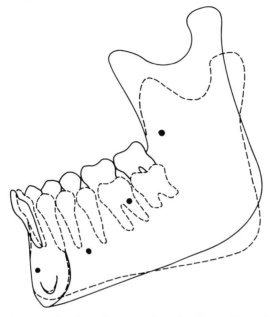

Fig. 17.1 *Diagram showing the mesial path of eruption of mandibular posterior teeth. The solid lines indicate the growth.*

These include mechanisms such as the mesial component of the occlusal force, and the mesial component of the path of eruption of the mandibular posterior teeth (Fig. 17.1). It has also been suggested that crowded posterior teeth drive the buccal segments mesially in their attempts to erupt, but as yet there is no strong evidence to support this view.

The Crowns of the Mandibular Anterior Teeth Moving Lingually

In boys, mandibular incisors become more upright at adolescence. This appears to be related directly to an increase in mandibular prognathism. Some workers have suggested that the mandibular incisor roots are carried forward by growth while the crowns are restrained by occlusal contact against the upper incisors. Others believe that this restraining effect is provided by the lip musculature. Recently, however, doubt has been cast on this uprighting effect as a cause of late crowding[4].

Narrowing of the Mandibular Arch

This widely recognised and well-documented change in the canine region appears to take place throughout life. The cause is unknown.

PRESENTATION WITH LATE CROWDING

Upon review at 16 or 17 years of age, patients often express disproportionate concern about minimal changes in mandibular incisor crowding. This is particularly so where fixed appliance techniques have produced perfect incisor alignment which then relapses to some extent following removal of retaining appliances. Concern includes one or more of the following:

- will it get worse?
- how much worse will it get?
- for how long will it go on worsening?
- will it interfere with oral hygiene?

It is now being recognised that it is very important for the orthodontist to explain to patients who are about to embark on orthodontic treatment that while appliances may enable the teeth to be fully aligned, it is almost certain that there will be some degree of post-treatment relapse, and that in some cases a very marked deterioration will take place, once appliances are withdrawn. It is equally important for the general dentist to realise that this will be the case; he or she should be sympathetic to the problem and certainly not heighten the patient's anxiety by drawing attention to minor post-treatment changes when these are observed.

The extent to which any crowding (be it post-treatment or arising *de novo*) will go on worsening is always extremely difficult to predict; estimates can generally be little more than guesses. Even if the patient's growth in stature has ceased, active facial growth may still be taking place, indeed peak rates of facial growth can follow those of height by as much as 3 years[5]. However, generally changes in the rate of facial growth follow those of stature[6], and significant changes in mandibular arch crowding are unusual after this time (Figs. 17.2; 17.3*a* and *b*, p. 138).

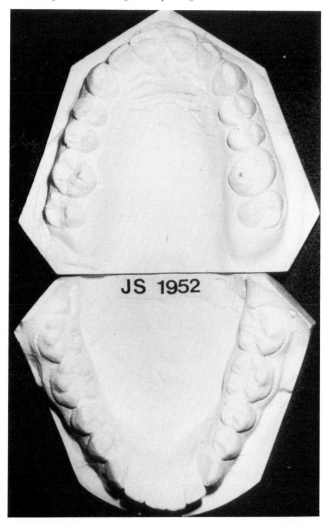

Fig. 17.2 *Study models of a patient with a Class I occlusion and almost perfect mandibular incisor alignment at the age of 25. Compare with Fig. 17.3.*

TREATMENT OF THE MANDIBULAR ARCH

Because of the inevitability of late teenage changes in the lower arch, some orthodontists now aim to leave 'safey valve' space distal to the mandibular canines at the completion of treatment.

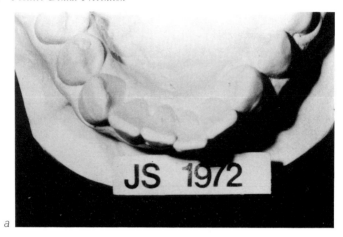

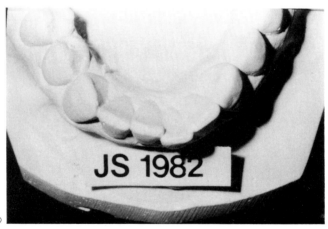

Fig. 17.3a and **b** *Models of the mandibular teeth of the patient in Fig. 17.2 showing: a = Late crowding at 45 years of age; b = Further deterioration by 55 years. The periodontal health is excellent.*

While this is relatively easy to achieve when premolars have been removed, it cannot readily be accomplished in other instances. Furthermore, if a satisfactory buccal occlusion is to remain, the presence of mandibular arch spacing must be matched by a similar space in the upper arch, and this may not be regarded with favour by the patient.

Patients with ideal occlusions who develop late crowding should be sympathetically reassured that this is entirely normal and told that, in the presence of good oral hygiene, it is of no dental significance. Such crowding should, however, be monitored by means of plaster models or photographs. Where the situation becomes stable, the clinician can then demonstrate after an elapse of several more months that no further change has taken place.

Where alignment continues to deteriorate, there are (apart from accepting this) several possibilities, none of which should be undertaken without first obtaining specialist advice.

Removal of Posterior Teeth to Reduce Mesial Migration

While the removal of third molars may be indicated on other grounds, this 'solution' cannot be justified on the basis of its effect on preserving mandibular arch alignment. Loss of third molars does not eliminate this risk; indeed, any effect is very marginal. Loss of the mandibular second molar, on the other hand, does appear to reduce the degree of late mandibular incisor imbrication[7]. Unfortunately, it is not, as yet, possible to reliably distinguish (at 12–18 years of age) patients in which the mandibular third molars will erupt satisfactorily, and those in whom they will not. Hence loss of the second molar may result in a third molar which requires active alignment with fixed appliances.

Permanent Retention of the Mandibular Incisor Teeth

For the dentally conscious patient with excellent oral hygiene, the use of permanent retention of the mandibular anterior teeth can be justified. The placing of a bonded lingual wire is a quick, reliable and reversible procedure which is particularly appropriate when severe irregularity has required active treatment. In the absence of retention, such patients always show some degree of regression, even after prolonged retention. The use of retainers where no treatment has been necessary in the mandibular arch, or where the incisors achieved alignment spontaneously following extraction of premolars, is more debatable. In these situations it is more appropriate to monitor mandibular arch alignment using reference models to ensure that any slight changes can be identified sufficiently early to allow the retainer option to be considered.

Interdental Reduction (Stripping) of Mandibular Anterior Teeth

This procedure, whereby abrasive strips and discs are used to reduce the mesial and distal surfaces of the teeth, may provide a rapid solution in certain selected cases but it has a number of inherent drawbacks. The amount of reduction possible is clearly very limited, and any space created may be quickly lost by further mesial migration of posterior teeth. Permanent retention may therefore be needed after the tooth positions have been corrected, particularly where the stripping is carried out early. Perhaps the greatest drawback to the method concerns the long-term prognosis of the teeth concerned. Especially where the lower incisors are of a rather tapering form, loss of crown width by interdental stripping can produce a loss of supporting bone at the interdental crest. One has to answer the question: 'would I rather have correctly shaped, but imbricated mandibular incisors to maintain in adult life, or would I be prepared to try to manage mandibular incisors that are well aligned but difficult to scale, etc., because they have been flattened mesially and distally?'

TREATMENT OF THE MAXILLARY ARCH

Treatment of the adult complaining of deteriorating alignment of maxillary incisor teeth should not be entered into lightly. Successful treatment will almost invariably require the use of fixed appliances in both arches and often permanent retention will also be necessary.

REFERENCES

1. Fastlicht J. (1970). Crowding of the lower incisors. *Amer. J. Orthod*; **58**: 157–63.
2. Steigman S., Weissberg Y. (1985). Spaced dentition: an epidemiologic study. *Angle Orthod*; **55**: 165–76.
3. Todd J. E., Walker A. M. (1983). *Adult dental health, England and Wales 1968–1978.* London: HMSO.
4. Richardson M. E. (1979). Late mandibular incisor crowding: facial growth or forward drift. *Europ. J. Orthod*; **1**: 219–25.

5. Bishara S. E., Jamison J. E., Peterson L. C., Dekock W. H. (1981). Longitudinal changes in the standing height and mandibular parameters between the ages of 8 and 17 years. *Amer. J. Orthod*; **80**: 115–35.
6. Ekstrom C. (1982). *Facial Growth Rate and its Relation to Somatic Maturation in Healthy Children.* Thesis. Stockholm: Karolinska Institute.
7. Richardson M. E. (1983). The effect of mandibular second molar extraction on late mandibular arch crowding. *Angle Orthod*; **53**: 25–8.

Index

Harvold Activator, 115 (Fig.), 117

immunological deficiency, 43
immunological response, 7
impacted first permanent molars,
   111
incisors
   accidental damage, 3; *see also*
      avulsed anterior tooth
   imbrication, 133, 134

Lactobacillus counts, 25
leukaemia, 43
lips, incompetent, 41

malocclusion, 29–38, 96, 141
   alignment of anterior teeth, 133
   early detection, 29–38
   interdental reduction
      (stripping) of anterior
      teeth, 140
   maxillary canines, misplaced,
      33
   narrowing of the mandibular
      arch, 136
   permanent retention of incisor
      teeth, 139
   presentation with late
      crowding, 136, 137 (Fig.),
      138 (Fig.)
   prevention after eruption of
      second permanent molars,
      133–41
      late crowding, 134–5
      narrowing of mandibular
         arch, 136
   reasons for eliminating, 29–30
   removal of posterior teeth, 139
metronidazole, 43
mixed dentition, occlusal
   assessment, 30–8, 96–113
mottling (enamel fluorosis), 55–6
mouthbreathing, 41
mouthguards, 122–3

myofunctional appliances, 114–21
   Class II division 2 incisor
      relationships, 119
   limitations, 119–21
   prevention, role in, 117–18
   prominent incisors, 118–19
   relevance of growth, 116–17
   severe skeletal Class II
      malocclusion, 119,
      120 (Fig.)

occlusal assessment in mixed
   dentition, 30–8, 96, 113
occlusion, 2
Oral Health Goals (WHO), 6, 22
oral hygiene, 6, 22, 49–50
   instruction, 39–45
orthodontic need, 6
orthodontics, 29–38, 96–141
orthopantomogram (OPG), 31, 32
   (Fig.), 37, 98 (Fig.), 99 (Fig.),
   100 (Fig.)
outline form, 66–7
overcutting, 67–8

periodontal attachment loss, 7
periodontal disease, 2, 7–13, 39–45
   advanced, children with, 2,
      12–13, 43–4
   antibiotic therapy, 43
   oral hygiene instruction, 39–41
   preventive management of,
      39–45
   screening for, 8–9
periodontal probe, 10
periodontal pocket, 8–11
periodontitis, juvenile, 8, 13
   chlorhexidine irrigation, 42
   treatment plan, 44
pit and fissure carious lesions,
   (Plates 2–3, 6–8)
   adolescents' control
      programme, 49–50
   chemical control, 42